Patricia P. Rosati, MS, RN, OCN

Student Workbook and Resource Guide for

Medical-Surgical Nursing Care

Third Edition

Karen M. Burke, RN, MS
Elaine L. Mohn-Brown, RN, EdD
Linda Eby, RN, MN

Pearson

Boston   Columbus   Indianapolis   New York   San Francisco   Upper Saddle River
Amsterdam   Cape Town   Dubai   London   Madrid   Milan   Munich   Paris   Montreal   Toronto
Delhi   Mexico City   Sao Paulo   Sydney   Hong Kong   Seoul   Singapore   Taipei   Tokyo

Pearson® is a registered trademark of Pearson plc

Pearson Education LTD.
Pearson Education Australia PTY, Limited
Pearson Education Singapore, Pte. Ltd
Pearson Education North Asia Ltd
Pearson Education, Canada, Ltd

Pearson Educación de Mexico, S.A. de C.V.
Pearson Education—Japan
Pearson Education Malaysia, Pte. Ltd
Pearson Education, Upper Saddle River, New Jersey

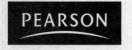

10 9 8 7 6 5 4 3 2 1
ISBN 10:   0-13-608011-1
ISBN 13: 978-0-13-608011-4

Contents

Preface

Students entering the field of nursing have a tremendous amount to learn in a very short time. This concise student workbook and resource guide has been developed to help you learn and apply key concepts and procedures, and master critical-thinking skills based on *Medical-Surgical Nursing Care*.

At the beginning of each chapter you will find an Explore MyNursingKit box. Just as in the main textbook, this box identifies some specific resources available at www.mynursingkit.com for the chapter. In addition, each chapter includes a variety of questions and activities to help you comprehend difficult concepts and reinforce basic knowledge gained from textbook reading assignments. Highlights of this workbook include:

- Chapters that correlate directly to *Medical-Surgical Nursing Care* to allow you to easily locate information related to each question.
- Thorough assessment of essential information in the chapter through generous use of multiple-choice and matching-style questions.
- Clinical case studies that provide scenarios to sharpen critical-thinking and clinical reasoning skills.
- Answers included in an appendix to provide immediate reinforcement and to allow you to check the accuracy of your work.

It is our hope that this workbook contributes to your success in the exciting and challenging field of medical-surgical nursing care.

Patricia P. Rosati, MS, RN, OCN
Allied Medical and Technical Institute
Scranton, PA

Chapter 1

Nursing in the 21st Century

KEY TERMS

Match each term with its appropriate definition.

H	1. Client-centered care	A.	Concerned with the whole person—physical, emotional, spiritual aspects
C	2. Caregivers	B.	First phase of the nursing process
J	3. Advocate	C.	People who provide personal assistance
A	4. Holistic	D.	Conclusion about a client's health status
B	5. Assessment	E.	Use of cognitive knowledge to choose best action
D	6. Nursing diagnosis	F.	Criterion to measure quality of practice
I	7. Outcomes	G.	Harm that results through actions of a licensed person
E	8. Critical thinking	H.	Care focused on uniqueness of the individual
F	9. Standard	I.	Achievable, measurable goals
G	10. Malpractice	J.	One who speaks for another and promotes client's rights

LEARNING OUTCOMES

1. What is medical-surgical nursing?

2. Identify some Healthy People 2020 Leading Health Indicators.

3. What is quality assurance?

4. What are some objectives of an advocate?

5. List the phases of the nursing process.

6. What is critical thinking?

7. Name six components regarding the LPN/LVN Scope of Practice.

8. What is the purpose of HIPAA?

9. Define ethics.

10. What are professional boundaries?

APPLY WHAT YOU LEARNED

The student nurses are beginning to study the nursing process. The students understand that the process is individualized and begins with data collection.

1. Describe the phases of the nursing process.

2. What happens during the evaluation phase?

3. How is a nursing diagnosis different from a medical diagnosis?

MULTIPLE CHOICE

Circle the answer that best completes the following statements.

1. A choice between two unpleasant alternatives is known as:
   A. ethics.
   B. assessment.
   C. dilemma.
   D. evaluation.

2. The ethical principle that involves the nurse doing no harm to clients is:
   A. beneficence.
   B. autonomy.
   C. accountability.
   D. nonmaleficence.

3. Purposeful actions to meet physical, psychosocial, and cultural needs of clients are:
   A. interventions.
   B. quality assurance.
   C. nursing diagnosis.
   D. implementation.

4. Nursing that is concerned with the whole person—physical, emotional, and spiritual—is:
   A. medical.
   B. psychological.
   C. ethical.
   D. holistic.

5. The nurse is teaching the client about a medication that has just been prescribed. Review of side effects and length of treatment has the client concerned. The nurse knows that giving the client this information to make decisions regarding care makes the nurse an:
   A. ethics committee member.
   B. advocate.
   C. implementation specialist.
   D. identifier of data.

6. Medical information that is obtained through observation or measurement is known as:
   A. objective.
   B. subjective.
   C. data.
   D. focused.

7. The nurse recognizes that designing interventions and outcomes is part of which phase of the nursing process?
   A. Diagnosis
   B. Implementation
   C. Assessment
   D. Planning

8. Determining whether the plan was effective or needs to be revised is completed during the:
   A. evaluation.
   B. implementation.
   C. planning.
   D. assessing.

9. Recognizing a pattern or clinical situation and combining it with knowledge and previous experience is known as:
   A. empathy.
   B. discipline.
   C. intuition.
   D. intellectual courage.

10. Laws that limit nursing practice to those licensed and practicing as nurses within a state are known as:
    A. scope of practice.
    B. statutory law.
    C. regulatory law.
    D. administrative law.

11. The nurse going to the cafeteria with friends begins to tell them about a new client. The nurse says that he is the mother's neighbor and continues to discuss his medical care. The nurse should understand that this is a violation of:
    A. ethics.
    B. malpractice.
    C. HIPAA.
    D. standards.

12. When a nurse administers a medication against the will of a mentally competent client, it is known as:
    A. battery.
    B. assault.
    C. defamation.
    D. false imprisonment.

13. Management and using data, information, and knowledge through computer information systems is:
    A. quality assurance.
    B. risk management.
    C. digital medicine.
    D. healthcare informatics.

14. The phase that includes a thorough history and physical assessment is:
    A. initial assessment.
    B. objective data.
    C. subjective data.
    D. focused assessment.

15. The nurse understands that using knowledge, experience, understanding, values, and ability to identify options is part of which process?
    A. Ethical dilemmas
    B. Clinical reasoning
    C. Intuition
    D. Clinical delegation

Chapter 2

Health, Illness, and Settings of Care

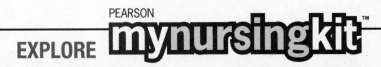

EXPLORE **PEARSON mynursingkit**™

MyNursingKit is your one stop for online chapter review materials and resources. Prepare for success with additional NCLEX®-style practice questions, interactive assignments and activities, web links, animations and videos, and more!

Register your access code from the front of your book at
www.mynursingkit.com

KEY TERMS

Match each term with its appropriate definition.

J___ 1. Health   A. Maintaining a dynamic steady state or balance

A___ 2. Homeostasis   B. Signs and symptoms

E___ 3. Disease   C. Disease that occurs rapidly and is self-limiting

B___ 4. Manifestations   D. Severity of illness and level of care required

I___ 5. Illness   E. Disruptions in structure and function of body or mind

C___ 6. Acute illness   F. Disease with unknown cause

H___ 7. Remission   G. Disease that exists at birth

D___ 8. Acuity   H. Period in which client is not experiencing symptoms even though disease is present

F___ 9. Idiopathic   I. Response a person has to a disease

G___ 10. Congenital   J. State of complete physical, mental, and social well-being

LEARNING OUTCOMES

1. What is the health–illness continuum?

2. What is homeostasis?

3. What is illness?

4. Name five characteristics of a chronic illness.

5. What is long-term care?

6. What is community-based nursing?

7. Name eight or more community-based nursing care settings.

8. What clients benefit from home healthcare services?

9. List safety concerns a home health nurse should assess.

10. Name five suggestions for effective home care.

APPLY WHAT YOU LEARNED

The nurse is assigned to care for a 72-year-old client who has been experiencing falls and some cognitive issues. Upon entering the client's home, the nurse notices that the bathroom is on the second floor and the house appears dark and poorly lit.

1. What safety issues should the nurse teach the client?

2. What community resources could the nurse recommend?

MULTIPLE CHOICE

Circle the answer that best completes the following statements.

1. The body's tendency to maintain a dynamic steady state or balance under constantly changing conditions is:
   - ✓ A. homeostasis.
   - B. disease.
   - C. illness.
   - D. wellness.

2. A disease that results from changes in the internal environment is known as:
   - A. toxic.
   - B. environmental.
   - C. lifestyle.
   - ✓ D. biological.

3. The nurse understands that the purpose of community-based care is to provide direct services to individuals to manage health problems and promote:
   - A. nursing.
   - B. medicine.
   - C. physicians.
   - ✓ D. self-care.

4. The process of learning to live to one's maximum potential with a chronic impairment and the resulting functional disability is known as:
   - A. long-term care.
   - B. disability.
   - ✓ C. rehabilitation.
   - D. cognitive therapy.

5. The nurse is caring for a client who presents with pain, nausea, and anxiety. These are known as:
   - A. assessments.
   - B. stressors.
   - ✓ C. manifestations.
   - D. disease.

6. A client has been undergoing testing for complaints of abdominal pain. All tests have come back negative and the client is still experiencing pain. The nurse knows the class of disease with an unknown cause is known as:
   - A. congenital.
   - B. psychosomatic.
   - C. iatrogenic.
   - ✓ D. idiopathic.

7. A period of time where symptoms reappear during an illness is:
   - ✓ A. exacerbation.
   - B. remission.
   - C. end stage.
   - D. acute.

8. The severity of the client's illness and the level of care required is referred to as:
   A. illness.
   B. acuity. ✔
   C. disease.
   D. health care continuum.

9. The nurse is doing a home evaluation for a 72-year-old client who lives alone. What would indicate an intervention by the nurse?
   A. Current medications
   B. Inadequate food supply ✔
   C. Absence of throw rugs
   D. Open blinds

10. The purpose of the nursing assessment visit is to:
    A. formulate a diagnosis for the physician.
    B. submit to Medicare.
    C. refer to the nursing home.
    D. identify client's needs. ✔

11. The nurse understands that all of the following are community-based nursing care settings except:
    A. mental health centers.
    B. senior centers.
    C. hospitals. ✔
    D. free clinics.

12. A nurse who helps bridge gaps between members of the church and the healthcare system is involved in:
    A. mental health nursing.
    B. home health nursing.
    C. forensic nursing.
    D. parish nursing. ✔

13. The degree of observable and measurable impairment is:
    A. impairment.
    B. handicap.
    C. rehabilitation.
    D. disability. ✔

14. A chronic illness is characterized by all of the following except:
    A. it is permanent.
    B. leaves a disability.
    C. it is reversible. ✔
    D. requires long periods of care.

15. The nurse understands that an acute illness is:
    A. non-reversible.
    B. self-limiting. ✔
    C. malignant.
    D. congenital.

Chapter 3

Cultural and Developmental Considerations for Adults

KEY TERMS

Match each term with its appropriate definition.

C	1.	Culture	A.	Area surrounding one's body
J	2.	Race	B.	Change from the normal health state
A	3.	Personal space	C.	Learned behavior started by a group of people
B	4.	Alterations in health	D.	Group of people who share backgrounds such as religion or residence
I	5.	Family	E.	Peoples' beliefs that their values are the only acceptable ones
D	6.	Ethnic group	F.	Multigenerational family unit, including all relatives
K	7.	Ethnocentrism	G.	Roles and relationships of family members
H	8.	Nuclear family	H.	Man, woman, and biological children
G	9.	Family structure	I.	Unit of people related by marriage, birth, or adoption
F	10.	Extended families	J.	Differences in physical characteristics, such as skin color and eye shape

LEARNING OUTCOMES

1. Name five components of culture.

2. What are health disparities?

3. What special care considerations are there for Jehovah's Witnesses?

4. List health risks for young adults.

5. What are the tasks of a family?

6. What is ethnocentrism?

7. List the components of communication.

8. What importance does personal space have?

9. What is social orientation?

10. Identify some health risks for middle adults.

APPLY WHAT YOU LEARNED

The student nurse is speaking with high school students regarding growth and development. Some students tell her that they have one father and a stepmother while other students report having lived with grandparents, or two mothers.

1. What types of family structures are represented?

2. What types of health promotion could be taught to these students?

MULTIPLE CHOICE

Circle the answer that best completes the following statements.

1. A group of people who share experiences and backgrounds based on status, religion, and residence are known as:
    A. cultural groups.
    B. race groups.
    C. social groups.
    ✓ D. ethnic groups.

2. The nurse knows that the middle adult is within the age range of:
    A. 65–85.
    B. 35–65.
    C. 25–55.
    ✓ D. 40–65.

3. When speaking to a group of women between 18–40, the nurse knows the importance of a clinical breast exam and mammography at least every:
    ✓ A. 3 years.
    B. 5 years.
    C. 1 year.
    D. 2 years.

4. The number of Asian Americans is predicted to double by 2021 along with which group?
    A. Japanese
    ✓ B. Hispanics
    C. Mid-Atlantics
    D. Africans

5. The nurse is teaching the client about personal space. Knowing this client is from Canada means that they require:
    ✓ A. more personal space.
    B. less personal space.
    C. no personal space.
    D. eye contact only.

6. A Roman Catholic client is having their first post-op meal on Friday and the nurse is helping them select their menu. Considering Lent, which food should be avoided?
    A. Broccoli
    B. Milk
    ✓ C. Meat
    D. Fish

7. In order to give the most culturally competent care, the nurse must be aware of:
    A. psychology.
    ✓ B. his or her own values.
    C. anatomy.
    D. physiology.

8. Temporal orientation means:
   A. sound judgment.
   B. balanced thoughts.
   ✓ C. orientation in time.
   D. future judgment.

9. Recognizing the denomination of Seventh-Day Adventist, the nurse needs to respect that this day is considered the Sabbath for them:
   A. Monday.
   ✓ B. Saturday.
   C. Sunday.
   D. Friday.

10. The nurse recognizes that the beginning of wrinkles, gray hair, slight decline in cardiac output, and some loss of visual acuity occurs starting in the:
    A. 20s.
    B. 40s.
    ✓ C. 30s.
    D. 50s.

11. The leading cause of injury and death in people between ages 15 and 24 is:
    ✓ A. accidents.
    B. suicide.
    C. occupational.
    D. homicides.

12. When considering the leading cause of death for those between the ages of 25 and 64, the nurse would know that it is:
    A. cardiac arrest.
    B. stroke.
    C. hypertension.
    ✓ D. cancer.

13. What degree of change in glucose tolerance occurs in the middle adult?
    A. None
    ✓ B. Gradual decrease
    C. Gradual increase
    D. Sudden decrease

14. A unit of people related by marriage, birth, or adoption is called a:
    ✓ A. family.
    B. culture.
    C. ethnic group.
    D. race.

15. The nurse understands that by promoting health in adult clients through education, he or she is also promoting:
    A. nursing.
    B. community.
    ✓ C. wellness.
    D. faith.

Chapter 4

The Older Adult in Health and Illness

KEY TERMS

Match each term with its appropriate definition.

J 1. Aging

C 2. Free radicals

E 3. Apoptosis

A 4. Havighurst

G 5. Ageism

B 6. Dementia

D 7. Erikson

H 8. Senescence theory

I 9. Sundowning

F 10. Kohlberg

A. Believed the major tasks of old age centered on maintaining social contacts and relationships

B. Term used to refer to different kinds of organic disorders that progressively affect cognitive function

C. Unstable and reactive molecules

D. Identified ego integrity versus despair and disgust as the last stage of human development

E. Normal process occurring in cellular death

F. Believed older adults have completed the stages of moral development, and are at the conventional level

G. Form of prejudice against older adults

H. Premise that focuses on why people live as long as they do

I. Confusion that occurs after dark

J. Universal process beginning at birth

LEARNING OUTCOMES

1. Define ageism and list two myths about older adults.

2. What is gerontologic nursing and what is the projected future of this trend?

3. Discuss the term cognition and list some examples pertaining to the older adult.

4. Which developmental stage does Erikson identify for the older adult?

5. How would the nurse encourage reminiscence in the older adult?

6. What are some age-related physical changes in the older adult?

7. What is meant by psychosocial change? List some examples.

8. How would the nurse teach the older adult about prevention of accidents?

9. What is Alzheimer's disease?

10. How would the nurse describe methods to improve/maintain an older adult's quality of life?

APPLY WHAT YOU LEARNED

You are working with a client who is about to be discharged from the hospital after a fall. She will be returning to her home where she lives alone. She is 68 years old and takes medication only for hypertension. Her family is present at the time of discharge and tells you that they will stop over and check on her periodically.

1. What are some teaching points you can give to the client and family about preventing accidents in the home?

2. What are some concepts that will assist in health promotion of the older adult?

3. Would you request other disciplines to see her? If so, why?

MULTIPLE CHOICE

Circle the answer that best completes the following statements.

1. The nurse overhears a 76-year-old client's family member state, "Well he's had his good years. What can he possibly do to help us when he gets out?" This is a form of:
   A. genetic theory.
   B. apoptosis.
   ✓C. ageism.
   D. senescence.

2. Calcium intake in older adults should average:
   ✓A. 1200 mg per day.
   B. 600 mg per day.
   C. 800 mg per day.
   D. 1600 mg per day.

3. Older people continue to develop:
   A. judgmentally.
   ✓B. cognitively.
   C. gerontonlogically.
   D. accidentally.

4. You are assessing the physical condition of an 80-year-old male. You will not be surprised to find which of these signs and symptoms?
   A. Rales
   ✓B. Decreased skin turgor
   C. Smooth skin
   D. Visual acuity of 20/20

5. When making a home visit to your 66-year-old client, she states, "I made fried chicken and a peach cobbler yesterday. Would you care for some?" Your best reply should be:
   A. "Oh, no, that's too much fat!"
   B. "Sure, where is the butter?"
   ✓C. "I will send a dietician to discuss alternative cooking options."
   D. "Did you make collard greens also?"

6. The nurse is teaching the daughter of an elderly client about the aging process. The nurse would be correct if she stated:
   ✓A. "Your father may develop an enlarged prostate."
   B. "Estrogen levels begin to increase in females as they get older."
   C. "Hypoglycemia is common in the elderly."
   D. "The infection risks are decreased due to the adrenal gland's enlargement."

7. Which of the following conditions would most likely be seen in the older adult?
   ✓A. Cataracts
   B. Hypertension
   C. Herpes
   D. Obesity

8. You are talking to a client's son about the care his 78-year-old father will need at home. Your greatest concern for this client should be:
   A. Risk for Falls.
   B. Risk for Infection.
   C. Risk for Impaired Mobility.
   ✓D. Risk for Caregiver Role Strain.

9. The nurse is aware that a family who takes care of a client with Alzheimer's:
   A. realizes the disease is reversible.
   B. allows the client to wander without constraint.
   ✓C. may need the help of a support group.
   D. provides a stimulating environment.

10. Illness and loss of independence are:
    A. an expected part of the aging process.
    ✓B. not inevitable.
    C. government issues.
    D. all of the above.

11. Depression is often confused with:
    A. confusion.
    B. seizures.
    ✓C. dementia.
    D. dehydration.

12. When evaluating the nutritional status of an older client, the nurse should be aware of:
    A. exercise routine.
    B. environmental factors.
    ✓C. lost or damaged teeth/dentures.
    D. fiber intake.

13. The nurse knows that which of the following increases the risk of injury or illness in the older adult:
    A. widowhood.
    B. retirement.
    C. recreational activities.
    ✓ D. elder abuse.

14. In understanding the genitourinary system of the older adult, the nurse knows:
    A. kidneys increase in mass.
    ✓ B. kidneys decrease in mass.
    C. micturition reflex is increased.
    D. bladder capacity increases.

15. In order to assist the older adult in reminiscence, the nurse would:
    ✓ A. ask open-ended questions.
    B. ask yes/no questions so as to not confuse them.
    C. ask them to remember numerous details.
    D. ask them about painful memories.

Chapter 5

Guidelines for Client Assessment

KEY TERMS

Match each term with its appropriate definition.

D	1. Inspection	A.	Signs; observable or measurable information
I	2. Palpation	B.	Tapping the body to produce sound waves
B	3. Percussion	C.	Client as information source
F	4. Auscultation	D.	Observing/looking carefully
E	5. Subjective data	E.	Symptoms experienced by the client
A	6. Objective data	F.	Listening to sounds using a stethoscope
C	7. Primary source	G.	Family, friends, or records as information sources
G	8. Secondary source	H.	Objective and subjective data associated with an illness
H	9. Manifestations	I.	Using the hands to touch and feel
J	10. LOC	J.	Level of consciousness

LEARNING OUTCOMES

1. What is the purpose of the client assessment?

2. What are differences between subjective and objective data?

3. List components in a health history.

4. List four methods of physical examination.

5. What are some age-related assessment findings in the older adult?

6. Describe the assessment of the pupils.

7. Compare bradycardia and tachycardia.

8. What is the amplitude of the pulse?

9. How does the nurse evaluate mental status?

10. What are key concepts in documenting accurately?

APPLY WHAT YOU LEARNED

A client presents to your clinic with complaints of general body aches, little joy in activities, and loss of appetite. You notice the client is wearing torn clothes and appears unkempt. Through initial conversation, you discover that the client is a 34-year-old recently unemployed male who has two children to support.

1. Based upon the scenario above, what type of data would be considered objective?

2. Could the nurse list subjective data based upon the above information?

3. What type of assessment would be the focus for the nurse?

MULTIPLE CHOICE

Circle the answer that best completes the following statements.

1. Poor turgor and dry mucous membranes would be an indication of:
    - ✓A. fluid volume deficit.
    - B. fluid volume excess.
    - C. normal fluid balance.
    - D. not enough data to evaluate.

2. A grating sound heard during chest auscultation may be:
    - A. crackles.
    - ✓B. pleural friction rub.
    - C. rhonchi.
    - D. wheezes.

3. Your client complains of difficulty breathing when attempting to lie down. After your respiratory assessment, you note in the medical record that the client has a history of:
    - A. eupnea.
    - B. apnea.
    - ✓C. orthopnea.
    - D. dyspnea.

4. After the assessment of the eyes, the nurse would not document:
    - A. equality.
    - B. shape.
    - C. reactivity.
    - ✓D. color of iris.

5. The normal pupillary response to accommodation is:
    - A. dilatation and divergence.
    - B. dilatation and convergence.
    - C. constriction and divergence.
    - ✓D. constriction and convergence.

6. The use of adequate lighting is most important during:
    - A. auscultation.
    - B. percussion.
    - C. palpation.
    - ✓D. inspection.

7. Ms. Lewis has a fractured tibia and fibula. The nurse is performing an assessment of her extremities. The purpose of the blanching test is to evaluate:
    - ✓A. peripheral circulation.
    - B. cardiac output.
    - C. peripheral pulses.
    - D. nutritional deficiencies.

8. The student nurse is performing a cardiac assessment. You indicate your knowledge of the thoracic structures by properly palpating the PMI:
    - A. directly over the sternum at the fourth rib.
    - ✓B. at the left midclavicular line, fifth intercostal space.
    - C. at the right midclavicular line, fourth intercostal space.
    - D. at the left midclavicular line, parallel to the axilla.

9. While assessing your client's lung fields, you hear popping sounds during inspiration at the base of the left lung. You would classify these findings as:
   A. crackles.
   B. rhonchi.
   C. wheezes.
   D. rubs.

10. An example of objective data would include:
    A. the client's description of the pain.
    B. radial pulse rate of 66 bpm.
    C. sensation of itching after a bee sting.
    D. headache resulting from photosensitivity.

11. A client states that he has had severe abdominal cramping for the last two hours. This type of data would be classified as an example of:
    A. subjective data.
    B. objective data.
    C. disputable data.
    D. personal data.

12. When assessing peripheral pulses, the nurse must compare both extremities. The elements of this assessment include:
    A. rate.
    B. rhythm.
    C. strength.
    D. all of the above.

13. The nurse prepares to assess the client's abdomen. The correct order of assessment should be:
    A. inspection, auscultation, palpation.
    B. inspection, palpation, auscultation.
    C. auscultation, inspection, palpation.
    D. any order is acceptable.

14. Mr. Hibbard has been admitted to the orthopedic unit following a motor vehicle collision. Both arms are placed in long-arm casts. When taking the vital signs, the nurse must assess the pulse rate by:
    A. listening to the apical pulse for one full minute.
    B. placing the client on a cardiac monitor.
    C. checking the carotid pulses.
    D. not assessing the radial pulses due to location of the cast.

15. The most accurate method for assessing the pulse rate is:
    A. simultaneous bilateral manipulation of the carotid arteries.
    B. auscultating directly over the point of maximum impulse.
    C. palpating the radial pulses.
    D. auscultating the femoral pulses.

Chapter 6

Essential Nursing Pharmacology

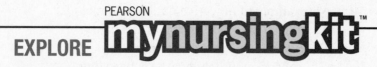

EXPLORE PEARSON mynursingkit™

MyNursingKit is your one stop for online chapter review materials and resources. Prepare for success with additional NCLEX®-style practice questions, interactive assignments and activities, web links, animations and videos, and more!

Register your access code from the front of your book at **www.mynursingkit.com**

KEY TERMS

Match each term with its appropriate definition.

B	1. Pharmacology	A.	Positioning or oral medication in the inner lining of the cheeks
J	2. Pharmacokinetics	B.	The study of drugs and their uses in the body
H	3. Absorption	C.	The process by which the body changes a drug from its original chemical structure to a form that can be readily eliminated or excreted
A	4. Buccal	D.	Injectable (drugs)
D	5. Parenteral	E.	Drug that prevents a receptor response or blocks a normal cellular response
E	6. Distribution	F.	Occurs after the drug has absorbed into the system
C	7. Metabolism	G.	The process by which drugs are eliminated from the body
G	8. Excretion	H.	The first step in the passage of a drug through the body
E	9. Antagonist	I.	The amount of time needed for elimination processes to decrease the original blood concentration by 50%
I	10. Half-life	J.	The study of how drugs are processed by the body

LEARNING OUTCOMES

1. What are the six rights of medication administration?

2. Describe the process of absorption and excretion in pharmacology.

3. What are the four names given to drugs?

4. What is the purpose of a loading dose?

5. Identify the differences between an idiosyncratic effect and a toxic effect.

6. Contrast agonist and antagonist drugs.

7. What is polypharmacy?

8. List some factors that affect drug responses.

9. Describe the concepts of synergism and potentiation.

10. List some factors to include in a medication history.

APPLY WHAT YOU LEARNED

You are caring for a 65-year-old male who tells you that he takes five prescription drugs and three over-the-counter medications that his physician is not aware he is taking. As the nurse, you begin to educate the client about the importance of reporting all medications to the doctor.

1. Describe some educational points the nurse will address with this client.

2. How the nurse will relay this information to the physician?

3. Discuss polypharmacy regarding this client.

MULTIPLE CHOICE

Circle the answer that best completes the following statements.

1. All healthcare facilities are required to have narcotic control systems in place (i.e., all narcotics are locked up). One way of insuring compliance is to:
   A. give narcotic keys to all employees.
   B. give narcotic keys to administrative staff only.
   C. give narcotic keys to authorized personnel.
   D. not enough data to evaluate.

2. The most widely used drug reference in the United States is:
   A. hospital formulary.
   B. *Facts and Comparisons.*
   C. PSA.
   D. PDR.

3. The absorption process occurs from the time a drug enters the body until:
   A. it reaches the site of action.
   B. half-life is achieved.
   C. excretion.
   D. it quits working.

4. Transdermal (applied to the skin) patches allow the body to absorb drugs slowly and usually:
   A. last longer.
   B. fall off easily.
   C. cause rashes.
   D. provide relief.

5. Intravenous drugs are delivered directly into the bloodstream and therefore:
   A. have the slowest excretion rate.
   B. have the fastest absorption rate.
   C. have the greatest half-life.
   D. have the longest duration of action.

6. The blood–brain barrier protects the central nervous system against severe toxic drug effects by preventing access to the:
   A. spinal fluid.
   B. cerebrospinal fluid. ✓
   C. synovial fluid.
   D. pleural cavity.

7. Drug metabolism refers to the process by which the body changes a drug from its original chemical structure to a form that can be readily eliminated or excreted. This is also called:
   A. biochemistry.
   B. bionics.
   C. biotransformation. ✓
   D. bioefficiency.

8. Drug toxicity in older adults occurs as a result of:
   A. ageism.
   B. negligence.
   C. confusion.
   D. polypharmacy. ✓

9. The effect of a drug depends on its:
   A. type and client.
   B. time and route.
   C. action and dose. ✓
   D. cost and manufacturer.

10. The nurse knows to include in her teaching:
    A. teas bind with tetracycline.
    B. a high carbohydrate diet decreases absorption of levodopa.
    C. a diet high in vitamin K reduces the effect of Coumadin. ✓
    D. a diet low in protein delays the effect of theophylline.

11. The usual adult dose of a drug is based upon which body weight?
    A. 200 lbs
    B. 100 kg
    C. 150 lbs ✓
    D. 150 kg

12. Over-the-counter (OTC) drugs account for what percentage of medication?
    A. 20%
    B. 60% ✓
    C. 50%
    D. 80%

13. What does the nurse check before administering any drug?
    A. Allergies ✓
    B. Likes and dislikes
    C. Side effects on the mother
    D. Insurance information

14. Which of these would not be included in a medication history?
    A. Allergies
    B. Use of OTC drugs
    C. Financial resources
    ✓ D. Employment status

15. What is the most important factor in administering medications to a 1-year-old infant?
    ✓ A. Weight of the child
    B. Age of the child
    C. Ethnicity of the child
    D. Sex of the child

Chapter 7

Caring for Clients With Altered Fluid, Electrolyte, or Acid–Base Balance

KEY TERMS

Match each term with its appropriate definition.

I	1. Thirst	A.	Primary regulator of water and electrolytes
H	2. Intracellular fluid	B.	Commonly caused by diarrhea or vomiting
C	3. Sodium	C.	Primary ECF cation
E	4. Extracellular fluid	D.	Higher concentration of solutes than plasma
D	5. Hypertonic	E.	Fluid found outside the cells
G	6. Osmolality	F.	Fluid found between the cells
F	7. Interstitial fluid	G.	Concentration of all solutes within body fluid
J	8. Potassium	H.	Fluid found inside the cells
A	9. Kidneys	I.	Primary indicator for regulation of water intake
B	10. Fluid volume deficit	J.	Primary ICF cation

LEARNING OUTCOMES

1. Contrast intracellular and extracellular fluid.

2. What are the vital functions of water in the body?

3. What is the purpose of electrolytes?

4. List components of body fluid regulation.

5. What are causes of fluid volume deficit?

6. What are causes of fluid volume excess?

7. Describe diagnostic testing to monitor fluid status.

8. List various IV solutions and their use.

9. Identify several high-sodium foods.

10. What is the effect of potassium on the body?

APPLY WHAT YOU LEARNED

Newly admitted 28-year-old female diagnosed with hypokalemia tells the nurse she drinks mostly water and tea and doesn't really eat solid foods. Her treatment plan will involve IV fluids and a nutritional consult. She will also have cardiac testing done.

1. What are some foods the dietician will recommend to this client?

2. According to the data above, would the nurse request any other consults?

3. What types of medication would the nurse expect to see ordered?

MULTIPLE CHOICE

Circle the answer that best completes the following statements.

1. The primary electrolyte that controls the water balance in the body is:
   - A. sodium.
   - B. potassium.
   - C. chloride.
   - D. magnesium.

2. Which of the following clients would be considered at greatest risk for dehydration?
   - A. Overweight male
   - B. Average-weight male
   - C. Underweight female
   - D. Overweight female

3. Of the following, which is not considered a function of an electrolyte?
   - A. Regulate acid–base balance
   - B. Needed for nutritional value
   - C. Maintain neuromuscular activity
   - D. Assist with enzyme reactions

4. Osmosis is the movement of:
   - A. particles across a semipermeable membrane.
   - B. water from an area of low-solute concentration to an area of higher concentration.
   - C. water and solutes across the capillary membranes.
   - D. solutes from an area of low concentration to an area of higher concentration.

5. Active transport is defined as:
   A. example of a sodium-potassium pump.
   B. the movement of molecules from an area of low-solute concentration to an area of high-solute concentration via the ATP mechanism.
   C. cells in a constant state of motion.
   D. molecules that continually move in and out of cells.

6. Mr. Smith has recently been diagnosed with a kidney dysfunction. He constantly complains of thirst. Which of the following statements to the client best indicates the nurse's understanding of the thirst mechanism?
   A. "Thirst is the primary regulator of water intake. When we are thirsty, we drink."
   B. "Thirst is important in maintaining fluid balance and preventing dehydration."
   C. "Thirst mechanisms decline with age, making the older adult at risk for dehydration."
   D. "A drop in blood volume stimulates the thirst center in the brain, which produces the sensation of 'thirst.'"

7. The mechanism of action for the antidiuretic hormone (ADH) may be defined as:
   A. kidneys reabsorb more water when the hormone is present.
   B. kidneys cease urine production when the hormone is present.
   C. blood osmolality increases as urine output decreases.
   D. the hypothalamus detects increased osmolality of the blood and stimulates the release of ADH.

8. The pathophysiology of SIADH is described as:
   A. a failure of the hypothalamus to release antidiuretic hormone.
   B. an excess of antidiuretic hormone in the bloodstream.
   C. water retention.
   D. copious amounts of concentrated urine.

9. Diabetes insipidus is caused by:
   A. failure of the hypothalamus to release antidiuretic hormone, resulting in excessive amounts of dilute urine.
   B. failure of the hypothalamus to release antidiuretic hormone, resulting in concentrated urine.
   C. failure of the pancreas to produce insulin, resulting in polyuria.
   D. total absence of antidiuretic hormone, resulting in severe water retention.

10. Alice is a 2-year-old child who has been suffering from vomiting and diarrhea for three days. Temperature is 102°F and she appears lethargic and exhausted. Her mother reports that Alice has not been able to keep anything down. Based on this information, Alice's primary nursing diagnosis should be:
    A. Activity Intolerance.
    B. Deficient Fluid Volume.
    C. Altered Nutrition: Less than Body Requirements.
    D. Risk for Diarrhea.

11. Your client has been admitted for uncontrollable vomiting. The doctor has ordered a Foley catheter and an IV of $D_5 \frac{1}{2}$ NS at 75 mL/hr. After the Foley was inserted, the initial amount of urine obtained was 100 mL. The IV was successfully begun, but one hour later the client's Foley bag had only drained 50 mL. Your next action would be to:
    A. administer an antiemetic in an attempt to stop the loss of gastric fluid.
    B. call the doctor and report the low urine output.
    C. continue to monitor.
    D. encourage the client to increase PO fluids.

12. Which electrolyte is most readily excreted by the kidneys and will be lost even when other electrolytes are conserved?
    A. Potassium
    B. Sodium
    C. Magnesium
    D. Calcium

13. Which of the following statements is false regarding the acid–base balance system?
    A. Blood buffers react quickly but are limited.
    B. The respiratory system adjusts the acid–base balance by either slowing or increasing respirations.
    C. The renal system is the slowest of the systems but is responsible for long-term balance.
    D. When hydrogen ions and the pH in the blood increase, the result is acidosis.

14. A client suffering from metabolic acidosis is most likely to:
    A. experience an increase in the blood pH.
    B. develop tachypnea.
    C. recover slowly, due to the kidney's role in acid–base balance.
    D. be diagnosed with acute pneumonia.

15. Mr. Jacobs, who was diagnosed with COPD 5 years ago, has been using his oxygen at home via nasal cannula. The flow rate is set at 2 L/min. Mr. Jacobs' respirations are 28/min, and he complains of SOB after minimal exertion. His wife is concerned that the amount of oxygen is "too low." Your best response should be:
    A. "I can't change the flow rate without an order."
    B. "Okay, let's increase the flow rate to 6 L/min and see how he does."
    C. "Increasing his oxygen may actually cut off his respiratory center in the brain."
    D. "I'll call the doctor and let him know about your concerns."

Chapter 8

Caring for Clients in Pain

KEY TERMS

Match each term with its appropriate definition.

E   1. Pain   A. Drugs that can be given alone for moderate-to-severe pain

H   2. Analgesia   B. Seeking of drugs for nonmedical reasons

H   3. Perception   C. Amount of pain endured before seeking relief

A   4. Opioids   D. Patient-controlled analgesia

E   5. Pain threshold   E. Unpleasant sensory or emotional experience

I   6. Respiratory   F. Point at which a person recognizes pain
        depression

D   7. PCA   G. Antidote for opioids

B   8. Addiction   H. Processing of pain impulses in the brain

C   9. Pain tolerance   I. Major side effect of most narcotics

G 10. Narcan   J. Pain relief

LEARNING OUTCOMES

1. What is the difference between pain tolerance and pain threshold?

2. Contrast acute pain and chronic pain.

3. List several factors that affect client response to pain.

4. What is patient-controlled analgesia?

5. What subjective data might be gathered when completing a pain evaluation?

6. What objective data may be seen in clients with pain?

7. What are some misconceptions about pain management?

8. List several nursing interventions for chronic pain.

9. Name several methods of complementary therapy.

10. What are possible side effects of opioid analgesics?

APPLY WHAT YOU LEARNED

A 37-year-old client is seen as a follow up for chronic back pain. She states her pain is a 7 on a 0–10 scale and she is out of medication. She was given a prescription for a 30-day supply two weeks ago. She then tells the nurse she has been laid off from her job and her rent is late.

1. How would the nurse question the client about the empty medication bottle?

2. What subjective and objective findings would the nurse expect to find in this client with a pain rating of "7"?

3. What nonpharmacological interventions could the nurse give this client?

4. Should the nurse be concerned with addiction? Why or why not?

MULTIPLE CHOICE

Circle the answer that best completes the following statements.

1. Natalie, a 26-year-old college student, has been admitted to your unit for observation. She has recently been found frequently crying alone in her room. She admits that she is constantly tired and irritable. The medical history reveals that Natalie was injured in a car crash two years ago and that she has never fully recovered. Natalie states that her back never stops hurting. You suspect that this may be diagnosed as:
    A. chronic pain syndrome.
    B. acute pain syndrome.
    C. chronic malignant pain.
    D. psychosomatic pain.

2. The nurse is caring for a client who received multiple fractures and contusions from a fall five days ago. At 3:30 P.M., the nurse administers the pain medication that was ordered q.i.d. At 5:00 P.M., the client calls for more pain medication. The assessment shows a BP of 160/88 and a pulse of 100. The nurse checks the chart and discovers that the client has made constant requests for pain relief on the previous shift. The best response would be to:
    A. ignore the client, as it appears he may be addicted to the medication.
    B. call the physician and report the addiction.
    C. administer another dose at 7:00 P.M.
    D. notify the physician that the current medication may not be effective.

3. Mrs. Hamrick is recovering from knee replacement surgery. Her pain medication order reads as follows: Vicodin 5/500 mg tabs 2 PO q.i.d. prn pain. She is scheduled for physical therapy from 10:00 to 11:00 A.M. It is now 7:00 A.M. She has not received a tab since 3:00 A.M. You will expect to administer the medication:
   A. at 9:30 A.M.
   B. at 10:00 A.M.
   C. after she returns from therapy.
   D. as soon as she calls for the medication.

4. Timothy, a 10-year-old, has twisted his ankle playing baseball. His mom asks you what other methods could be used to control the pain if the ordered medication does not work. You suggest:
   A. bring Timothy back to the clinic.
   B. place ice packs on the ankle for 20 minutes at a time for 24 hours.
   C. double the medication dosage.
   D. place warm packs on the ankle continuously for 24 hours.

5. A 70-year-old client with a history of Parkinson's disease and arthritis has been placed on Darvocet N100 1 tab PO t.i.d. prn pain. Which of the following would be a priority nursing diagnosis?
   A. Constipation
   B. Disturbed Thought Processes
   C. Risk for Injury
   D. Activity intolerance

6. Your client requires discharge teaching regarding his pain medication, Demerol tabs. Which of the following would be considered your highest priority?
   A. Do not take with alcohol
   B. Constipation may occur
   C. Sleepiness is a common side effect
   D. Nausea can be decreased by taking with food

7. Mrs. Johnnie has been ordered a PCA pump for pain control after her colon surgery. She voices concern about the potential for overdosing. Your best reply would be:
   A. "Don't worry, that never happens."
   B. "The pump is preset and you will only be allowed to receive that amount."
   C. "I'll teach you to use the pump and regulate the amount that you get."
   D. "If you are worried about it, we can give you injections instead."

8. A client has been receiving a new pain medication every four hours as ordered. His wife is concerned that he is very sleepy all the time and may be overmedicated. Your best response would be:
   A. "It really is strange that he is that sleepy."
   B. "I'll call the doctor. Thanks for telling me."
   C. "It is not unexpected with a new pain medication. We are checking him every two hours."
   D. "If he doesn't wake up in four hours, we'll get the medication changed."

9. You receive a call from a client who has been on long-term pain medications. She is worried that the pharmacist gave her "cheap stuff" because it does not help her pain. The client may be developing:
   A. increased pain.
   B. tolerance to the medication.
   C. decreased pain tolerance.
   D. chronic pain.

10. Mrs. Wesley is at the doctor's office for a checkup. She asks you why the doctor would prescribe an antidepressant when she is complaining of pain. She says, "I'm not crazy, my back has just hurt for so long." You base your response on the fact that:
    A. antidepressants are capable of relieving many types of pain.
    B. pain can cause confusion.
    C. chronic pain can affect mood and sleep patterns.
    D. opioids work best when taken with other medications.

11. A 17-year-old boy was admitted to the emergency department for fractures received during a football game. He is moaning and crying. After watching you administer a shot of Demerol, the father asks, "Why is my son acting like a baby? He's never acted like this before when a bone was broken!" Your response is based on the fact that:
    A. everyone perceives pain differently.
    B. everyone has a different pain threshold.
    C. previous experiences with pain can affect future coping behaviors.
    D. all of the above.

12. The tool used to measure pain is called a:
    A. Pain Tolerance Guide.
    B. Pain Threshold Scale.
    C. Pain Conduction Tool.
    D. Pain Scale.

13. Increased blood pressure, dilated pupils, perspiration, and pallor are signs of:
    A. opiate overdose.
    B. acute pain.
    C. adverse effects of Demerol.
    D. chronic pain.

14. Chronic nonmalignant pain is:
    A. known as cancer pain.
    B. due to back pain.
    C. ongoing pain caused by non–life-threatening causes.
    D. ongoing pain caused by a malignant tumor.

15. Response to pain is affected by:
    A. family and cultural expectations.
    B. pain tolerance.
    C. past experiences with pain.
    D. all of the above.

Chapter 9

Caring for Clients With Inflammation and Infection

KEY TERMS

Match each term with its appropriate definition.

F 1. Macrophage

A. First line of defense against external organisms

I 2. Phagocytosis

B. Hairs that remove trapped microorganisms from respiratory tract

G 3. Lymphadenitis

C. Chemicals released by macrophages that cause fever

___ 4. Leukocytosis

D. Medications used to treat bacterial infection

A 5. Skin

E. Tissue that lines the inner surfaces of the mouth and nose

E 6. Mucous membranes

F. Large WBC that ingest microorganisms and dead tissue

B 7. Cilia

G. A systemic response to inflammation

D 8. Antibiotics

H. Increased WBC production

J 9. Pathogen

I. The ingestion of microorganisms and dead tissue

C 10. Endogenous pyrogens

J. Microorganisms that are capable of causing disease

LEARNING OUTCOMES

1. List several factors that would cause inflammation.

2. What are the steps in the inflammatory response?

3. What are manifestations of local inflammation?

4. What manifestations are associated with systemic inflammation?

5. Name the links in the chain of infection.

6. List several common infectious diseases.

7. What are risk factors for healthcare-associated (nosocomial) infections?

8. Identify several Standard Precaution guidelines.

9. What subjective data would be presented by a client with an infection?

10. What would objective data be in a client with an infection?

APPLY WHAT YOU LEARNED

You are caring for a resident recently admitted from a nursing home with a fever and urinary tract infection. The resident has an indwelling Foley catheter. The resident is confused and does not answer questions appropriately. You notice a skin tear on the lower extremity that has no apparent dressing.

1. What lab tests is the nurse expecting to see ordered by the physician?

2. Can the nurse obtain subjective data from this client? Why or why not?

3. What course of treatment would the nurse expect to be ordered?

MULTIPLE CHOICE

Circle the answer that best completes the following statements.

1. Edema to an injured or infected site is which step in the inflammatory response?
   A. Vascular
   B. Cellular
   C. Healing
   D. Chemical

2. Nursing interventions for a client with acute inflammation are aimed at which cardinal manifestations of inflammation?
   A. Redness, swelling, pain
   B. Warmth, pain, impaired function
   C. Swelling, impaired function, pain
   D. Redness, warmth, impaired function

3. You examine a WBC count ordered for a client. The WBC count is 3,000/mm^3. This value most likely indicates:
   A. leukocytosis, a bacterial infection.
   B. leukopenia, a viral infection.
   C. This is a normal WBC count.
   D. No information can be obtained from this value.

4. When interpreting a WBC differential, a "shift to the left" indicates which of the following?
   A. Large amount of immature WBCs, severe infection ✓
   B. Large amount of mature WBCs, severe infection
   C. Large amount of immature WBCs, cancer
   D. Large amount of mature WBCs, cancer

5. Cultures of blood, wounds, or other infected body fluids should be obtained:
   A. 30 minutes after the first dose of antimicrobial therapy.
   B. 24 hours after the first dose of antimicrobial therapy.
   C. 24 and 36 hours after the first dose of antimicrobial therapy.
   D. prior to beginning antimicrobial therapy. ✓

6. The nurse wears personal protective equipment (gloves, mask, gown, and goggles) to break which link in the chain of infection?
   A. Microorganism
   B. Reservoir
   C. Portal of exit
   D. Portal of entry ✓

7. Choose the nursing intervention that will break the chain of infection in a client with a contagious respiratory infection.
   A. Administer antibiotic therapy.
   B. Have all visitors wear a mask.
   C. Practice meticulous hand washing.
   D. All of the above. ✓

8. Which of the following microorganisms is easily transmitted from client to client on a nurse's hands?
   A. *Escherichia coli*
   B. *Staphylococcus aureus* ✓
   C. Streptococci
   D. Enterococcus

9. Inappropriate use of antibiotics contributes to healthcare-associated (nosocomial) infections because:
   A. some bacteria survive and become resistant to the antibiotic. ✓
   B. normal flora are killed.
   C. infections only occur in those people who are taking antibiotics.
   D. none of the above.

10. You are changing the linens for a client with a draining wound infected with MRSA. Which precautions should be taken?
    A. Wear gloves, gown, and mask to change linens
    B. Wear gloves to change linens
    C. Wear gloves and gown to change linens ✓
    D. No precautions are necessary

11. Which of the following clients is at the greatest risk of infection?
    A. 42-year-old client with a rib fracture
    B. 56-year-old client with enlarged prostate who drinks cranberry juice
    C. 62-year-old client with a history of TB exposure
    D. 76-year-old client with recent CVA and no flu vaccine ✓

12. Penicillin should be taken:
    - A. with food.
    - B. with yogurt.
    - ✓ C. with water.
    - D. until symptoms dissipate.

13. An example of a cephalosporin is:
    - ✓ A. cefazolin.
    - B. nafcillin.
    - C. potassium clavulanate.
    - D. gentamycin.

14. Clients requiring CDC Tier 2 Transmission-based Precautions have:
    - A. rare microorganisms transmitted by blood to any host.
    - ✓ B. virulent microorganisms easily transmittable to any host.
    - C. healthcare-associated (nosocomial) infections.
    - D. community-acquired infections.

15. You are caring for a hospitalized client who develops chickenpox after a visit from his 5-year-old son. Your client will require which level of precaution?
    - ✓ A. Negative air pressure room; visitors must wear a mask
    - B. Private room with visitors wearing a mask within 3 feet
    - C. Gown and gloves required if entering room
    - D. No precautions other than standard are necessary

Chapter 10

Caring for Clients Having Surgery

EXPLORE **PEARSON mynursingkit**™

MyNursingKit is your one stop for online chapter review materials and resources. Prepare for success with additional NCLEX®-style practice questions, interactive assignments and activities, web links, animations and videos, and more!

Register your access code from the front of your book at **www.mynursingkit.com**

KEY TERMS

Match each term with its appropriate definition.

E 1. Conscious sedation

J 2. General anesthesia

H 3. Postoperative phase

H 4. Emancipated minor

G 5. Dehiscence

C 6. Informed consent

F 7. Secondary intention

B 8. Regional anesthesia

A 9. Intraoperative phase

D 10. Evisceration

A. Period beginning with entry into the operating room

B. Local anesthesia

C. Operative permit

D. Protrusion of body organs from a wound

E. Provides analgesia/amnesia with wakefulness

F. Healing of a large, gaping, irregular wound

G. Separation of incisional wound

H. Person under age 18, lives independently

I. Period beginning with admittance to recovery area

J. Anesthesia that creates an unconscious state

LEARNING OUTCOMES

1. Contrast inpatient surgery and ambulatory surgery.

2. What must a perioperative nurse understand?

3. What are the components of informed consent?

4. List and describe three phases of the surgical experience.

5. What is the focus of preoperative care?

6. Describe nursing care on the day of surgery.

7. What happens in the body under anesthesia?

8. List several risk factors for deep venous thrombosis.

9. What is the difference between dehiscence and evisceration?

10. Discuss pain management for the postoperative client.

APPLY WHAT YOU LEARNED

You are caring for a postoperative client with a PCA for pain control. The client states they are not going to use it due to fear of addiction. They state that if the pain gets bad enough, they will ring for the nurse.

1. How would the nurse educate the client regarding the PCA pump?

2. Explain pain control in the postoperative client.

3. How would the nurse assess the client's readiness to use the PCA?

MULTIPLE CHOICE

Circle the answer that best completes the following statements.

1. The nurse should know that the client's surgery will be postponed if the hemoglobin level is below:
   A. 16 g per 100 mL.
   B. 10 g per 100 mL.
   C. 12 g per 100 mL.
   D. 14 g per 100 mL.

2. A diabetic client is more at risk for postoperative complications because:
   A. the prescribed diet cannot be consumed due to nausea.
   B. healing rarely takes place in the diabetic client.
   C. blood glucose levels can fluctuate uncontrollably.
   D. the client is unable to administer self-injections of insulin.

3. Preoperative medications must be administered:
   A. within 15 minutes of the ordered time.
   B. within 30 minutes of the ordered time.
   C. at the ordered time.
   D. after the skin scrub is completed.

4. While the surgical client is semiconscious and receiving IV therapy, the nurse should:
   A. keep the arms unrestrained so the joints will not stiffen.
   B. elevate the arm above the level of the heart.
   C. gently massage the arm to relieve muscle spasms and prevent clots from forming.
   D. monitor the IV site at frequent intervals.

5. Immediately following surgery, the client's vital signs must be checked every:
   A. 5 minutes.
   B. 15 minutes. ✓
   C. 20 minutes.
   D. 30 minutes.

6. Your client calls you to his room and tells you that something is wrong with his incision. You notice that the edges of the wound have separated and a small amount of beefy red tissue is observable. Your first response should be to:
   A. notify the physician.
   B. cover the wound with sterile dry dressing.
   C. place a normal saline sterile dressing over the wound. ✓
   D. ask the client how long ago this occurred.

7. The nurse will instruct the client receiving a local anesthetic that:
   A. no pain will be felt during the procedure.
   B. drowsiness is a side effect of the medication.
   C. bleeding is usually superficial. ✓
   D. consciousness will be lost.

8. The nurse should teach the client that, after surgery, DVT may be prevented by:
   A. raising the head of the bed.
   B. encouraging passive and active leg exercises. ✓
   C. keeping the knees elevated.
   D. encouraging coughing and deep breathing exercises.

9. Which of the following is at a greater risk for developing postsurgical and postanesthesia complications?
   A. 42-year-old scheduled for eye surgery
   B. 3-year-old scheduled for a hernia repair
   C. 80-year-old scheduled for a right hip replacement ✓
   D. 18-year-old scheduled for a cervical biopsy

10. You are asked to obtain an informed consent for a client who is scheduled for a bowel resection. Your main responsibility should be to:
    A. explain the risks involved with the surgery.
    B. discuss other medical options that might be useful for this client's condition.
    C. witness the client's signature of consent. ✓
    D. check the form for completeness.

11. Your client is scheduled for surgery in two hours. He asks you why the surgery has to be done right away. He insists on a detailed explanation of the procedure. The legal responsibility for explaining the procedure rests with the:
    A. charge nurse.
    B. hospital risk management team.
    C. physician who will perform the surgery. ✓
    D. patient advocate.

12. Coughing and deep breathing are techniques that must be taught to surgical patients to prevent:
    A. formation of clots at the incision site.
    B. lung collapse after the surgery.
    C. hypotension.
    D. prolonged pain.

13. Morphine and Demerol may be ordered as a preoperative medication to:
    A. eliminate spasms of the colon.
    B. enhance the effects of the anesthetic.
    C. decrease hypertensive episodes during surgery.
    D. reduce pain while in the recovery room.

14. It is important for the nurse to assess the client's home medications prior to surgery because:
    A. these medications may alter the client's perception of the surgery.
    B. the anesthetics received in the operative phase may cause toxicity of other drugs.
    C. some medications may interact with the anesthetics, causing undesired effects.
    D. routine medications are usually withheld the day of the surgery.

15. Mr. James is complaining of abdominal discomfort two days after his hernia repair. He tells you that he feels bloated and has no appetite. Your next action should be to:
    A. tell the client that this is normal and to ambulate as much as possible.
    B. ask Mr. James about his last bowel movement.
    C. assess bowel function.
    D. administer a stool softener.

Chapter 11

Caring for Clients With Altered Immunity

KEY TERMS

Match each term with its appropriate definition.

_E_ 1. Antigen

_C_ 2. Allergen

_G_ 3. Lymphoid system

_A_ 4. HLA

_H_ 5. Cell-mediated immunity

_B_ 6. Humoral immunity

_J_ 7. Natural immunity

_D_ 8. Acquired immunity

_I_ 9. Active immunity

_F_ 10. Passive immunity

A. Cell surface markers unique to each person

B. B cells that produce antibodies

C. Type of antigen responsible for allergic response

D. Artificially acquired immunity received as a result of a vaccination

E. Substance capable of producing an immune response

F. Antibodies received via the placenta

G. Main source of lymphocytes in the body

H. Protection mediated by helper and killer T cells

I. Memory cells are produced against specific antigens

J. Innate resistance to foreign substances

LEARNING OUTCOMES

1. What is the purpose of a leukocyte?

2. Identify the cells of the immune system.

3. What are the differences between IgG and IgA?

4. Contrast active and passive immunity.

5. List several recommended immunizations for adults.

6. What is anaphylaxis?

7. Describe four types of hypersensitivity reactions.

8. Name several natural rubber latex products.

9. What are autoimmune disorders?

10. List several manifestations of HIV infection.

APPLY WHAT YOU LEARNED

You are caring for a client who is newly diagnosed with HIV. There has been a positive diagnosis of Kaposi's sarcoma and upon visualization, there are white patches in the mouth. The client is a 28-year-old male and his partner is at the bedside trying to comfort him and help him to relax.

1. How would the nurse explain Kaposi's sarcoma to the client and his partner?

2. What are the white patches in the mouth of this client?

3. What nursing interventions can be done to assist the client and his partner regarding relaxation?

MULTIPLE CHOICE

Circle the answer that best completes the following statements.

1. The function of the bone marrow is to:
    A. mature lymphocytes into T cells.
    B. filter out damaged RBCs.
    ✓ C. manufacture blood cells.
    D. filter out foreign particles.

2. A nursing assistant tells the nurse that a rash is developing on her hands. The most appropriate response should be:
    A. "What are you washing your hands with?"
    B. "Don't wear any gloves when you give a bath."
    ✓ C. "Which type of gloves are you using?"
    D. "Do you have an allergy to peanuts?"

3. The nurse is providing teaching for a client scheduled for allergy skin testing. The client asks what kind of preparation is needed for the test. The best response might be:
    A. "You don't need to do anything."
    B. "Oh, I have to gather all the supplies for the doctor."
    C. "Nothing, but epinephrine will be given prior to the test."
    ✓ D. None of the above.

4. Adults should have a tetanus toxoid (Td) every:
   A. year.
   B. two years.
   C. five years.
   ✓ D. ten years.

5. The nurse is teaching a "safe-sex" class at a local high school. He knows that further teaching is necessary when one of the students states:
   ✓ A. "As long as I use a condom, I won't get anyone pregnant."
   B. "Wow, I didn't know that condoms should be made of latex."
   C. "I shouldn't have unprotected sex."
   D. "I guess that the condoms in my wallet are too old to use now."

6. You are assessing a client's immune status. Which of the following must be included in the documentation?
   ✓ A. Recent exposure to a friend with active tuberculosis
   B. Hernia repair four years ago
   C. Diagnosis of post-traumatic syndrome
   D. Low-pitched bowel sounds

7. You are preparing for the NCLEX-PN® by reviewing your immunology notes. Which of the following is not considered a part of the immune system?
   A. Thymus gland
   B. Appendix
   ✓ C. Gallbladder
   D. Spleen

8. A client has been taking diphenhydramine for hay fever symptoms. Which of the following is not a common side effect of the medication?
   A. Drowsiness
   B. Sedation
   ✓ C. Urinary retention
   D. Thirst

9. A client is taking cyclosporin to prevent rejection of his new kidney. The daily lab work is faxed to your unit. Which of the following would require a call to the physician?
   A. Glucose 93
   B. BUN 10
   ✓ C. WBC 3000
   D. Platelet count 150,000

10. You feel confident that your client, an organ transplant recipient, understands your discharge instructions when he says:
    ✓ A. "I'm going to take my temperature and weight at the same time every day."
    B. "I will take my Cellcept at the first sign of a fever."
    C. "As long as I don't drink after my children when they are sick, I am safe from infection."
    D. "I won't have to see my doctor unless I don't feel well."

11. Nursing care for any immunocompromised client includes removing invasive lines as soon as possible. The rationale for this intervention is that:
    A. the client can go home sooner.
    B. fewer sites are available for bacterial invasion.
    C. the client is more comfortable.
    D. signs of infection are easier to monitor.

12. Isolation precautions for the transplant client are designed to:
    A. reduce possible microorganisms transferred by the client.
    B. reduce possible microorganisms transferred to the client.
    C. reduce the risk of rejection.
    D. all of the above.

13. Your client, a 62-year-old female, has recently been diagnosed with rheumatoid arthritis. She tells you that she just doesn't feel like getting up in the mornings. Her housework is not getting done. An appropriate nursing diagnosis might be:
    A. Disturbed Body Image
    B. Fatigue
    C. Ineffective Individual Coping
    D. Acute Pain

14. In addition to the ELISA, which of the following tests is used to diagnose HIV?
    A. HIV viral load
    B. CD4 cell count
    C. Western blot
    D. All of the above

15. The appropriate statement to a client who admitted to "sharing a needle" should be:
    A. "If your HIV test is negative after three months, you have nothing to fear."
    B. "Don't worry, the HIV virus is only transmitted in semen."
    C. "Seroconversion usually occurs in six to twenty-four weeks."
    D. "Try not to think about it."

Chapter 12

Caring for Clients With Cancer

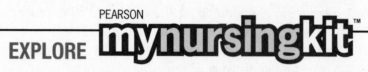

EXPLORE **mynursingkit**

MyNursingKit is your one stop for online chapter review materials and resources. Prepare for success with additional NCLEX®-style practice questions, interactive assignments and activities, web links, animations and videos, and more!

Register your access code from the front of your book at **www.mynursingkit.com**

KEY TERMS

Match each term with its appropriate definition.

E 1. Cancer   A. Process of invading other tissues
D 2. Oncologist   B. White blood cells
G 3. Neoplasm   C. Genes that can convert normal cells into cancer cells
A 4. Metastasis   D. Cancer specialist
C 5. Oncogenes   E. Group of neoplastic diseases
B 6. Lymphocytes   F. Effect of cancer cells on metabolism
F 7. Anorexia-cachexia   G. Any new abnormal growth
       syndrome
J 8. Classification   H. Cancer-causing agents
H 9. Carcinogens   I. Biochemical indicator of malignancy
I 10. Tumor markers   J. Naming of tumor tissue or cell of origin

LEARNING OUTCOMES

1. Contrast benign and malignant neoplasms.

2. What is an oncogene?

3. Name several controllable risk factors associated with cancer.

4. List some carcinogens associated with cancer.

5. What are possible cancer warning signs?

6. List several common general manifestations of cancer.

7. What is anorexia-cachexia syndrome?

8. Describe the tumor classification system.

9. List several oncologic emergencies.

10. What are common side effects of chemotherapy?

APPLY WHAT YOU LEARNED

A 65-year-old male was just admitted to your unit with anorexia related to prostate cancer with metastasis to the lungs. Consults have been ordered for dietary and hospice. His wife is at the bedside trying to engage him in conversation about anything other than cancer. He is staring blankly out of the window.

1. What interventions could the nurse use regarding the anorexia?

2. How would the nurse assist the client and his wife with his grieving?

3. What role will hospice nurses play in the care of this client?

MULTIPLE CHOICE

Circle the answer that best completes the following statements.

1. Nurses are aware that the second-leading cause of death in people over the age of 65 is:
   A. chronic obstructive pulmonary disease.
   B. end-stage renal failure.
   C. cancer.
   D. coronary artery disease.

2. You are teaching a health class at a local retirement center. When discussing the potential for prostate cancer in the older male, you include the following teaching point:
   A. Prostate self-examination every week
   B. X-ray of the prostate gland after the age of 65
   C. Screening for the presence of PSA
   D. CT scan of the chest to rule out metastasis

3. Mrs. Jackson has been diagnosed with breast cancer and metastasis to the spinal cord. She is paralyzed from the waist down and requires assistance with ADLs. Which of the following nursing diagnoses would be the most appropriate at this time?
   A. Risk for Infection
   B. Risk for Impaired Skin Integrity
   C. Risk for Injury
   D. Risk for Caregiver Role Strain

4. A divorced mother of four school-aged children is hospitalized with inoperable brain cancer. The client voices concern over the care for her children after her death. The best response should be:
   A. "You are going to live for a while longer and will have time to make arrangements."
   B. "Won't your ex-husband care for his kids after your death?"
   C. "I wouldn't worry about that right now. Just focus on getting well."
   D. "Would you like to share your thoughts with me?"

5. Interleukin-2 is used as therapy for a client with metastatic renal cancer. The nurse recognizes that the goal of this type of treatment might be:
   A. selectively altering the DNA of malignant cells.
   B. enhancing the client's immunologic response to tumor cells.
   C. stimulating malignant cells to enter mitosis.
   D. preventing bone marrow depression.

6. After the implantation of a radioactive cervical implant in an outpatient clinic, it is important to teach the client to:
   A. avoid close contact with others.
   B. limit activity to 30 minutes per day.
   C. eat three nutritious meals every day.
   D. dispose of the implant in the trash if it becomes dislodged.

7. You are reviewing a client's history prior to assisting in the development of a nursing care plan. You note that the client has been diagnosed with colon carcinoma. The staging classification is T_{IS}. You understand that this represents:
   A. a tumor with no metastasis.
   B. no evidence of a primary tumor.
   C. a tumor that is localized and encapsulated.
   D. two abnormal lymph nodes.

8. Several cancer warning signals have been identified. If all of the following are true, which signal would be particularly important to the chronic smoker?
   A. Obvious change in mole or wart
   B. A sore that does not heal
   C. Nagging cough
   D. Change in bowel habit

9. The nurse has completed a physical assessment on a client diagnosed with pancreatic cancer. Which of these findings indicates poor nutritional status?
   A. Positive muscle tone
   B. Good skin turgor
   C. Moist oral membranes
   D. Distended abdomen

10. A gastric cancer client is receiving high doses of 5-FU. Based on your knowledge of the side effects of this chemotherapy drug, which nursing intervention should take priority in the client's care?
    A. Six small meals a day
    B. Increase PO fluids
    C. Assess lungs for coarse rales
    D. Monitor lab values for the presence of uric acid

11. The drug tamoxifen is generally used in the treatment of:
    A. breast cancer.
    B. prostate cancer.
    C. small-cell lung cancer.
    D. bladder cancer.

12. A client who is being treated on an outpatient basis for kidney cancer telephones the nurse on duty and states, "I just don't think I can take any more treatments." The best response of the nurse should be:
    A. "Okay, I'll let your doctor know right away."
    B. "You sound terrible, what's the matter?"
    C. "Would you like to talk about your concerns?"
    D. "Please tell me your concerns."

13. Which of the following are not characteristics of a malignant neoplasm?
    A. Rapid growth
    ✓ B. Well-defined borders
    C. Noncohesive
    D. Invasive

14. The nurse is teaching the client about the care of radiation skin markings. Of the following, which should be most emphasized during the session?
    A. Protect the skin from sunlight.
    ✓ B. Do not wash off the markings.
    C. Do not apply heat or cold to the marked areas.
    D. Wear loose clothing.

15. The tool of choice for diagnosing head and neck cancer is:
    ✓ A. MRI.
    B. CT scan.
    C. x-ray imaging.
    D. ultrasonography.

Chapter 13

Loss, Grief, and End-of-Life Care

KEY TERMS

Match each term with its appropriate definition.

H 1. Loss
E 2. Grief
A 3. Death
C 4. Advance directives
G 5. Durable power of attorney
B 6. Living will
D 7. Comfort measures only order
F 8. Involuntary euthanasia
I 9. Hospice
J 10. DNR

A. Irreversible cessation of brain function
B. Personal expression of desires for end-of-life interventions
C. Planning for health care/financial matters in the event of incapacitation
D. Order indicating no life-sustaining measures; providing only soothing interventions at end of life
E. Emotional response to loss
F. Mercy killing
G. Transfer of power to another person for decisions in care
H. Absence or potential absence of a valued object, person, body part, or situation that was normally present
I. Model for end-of-life care in the face of limited life expectancy
J. Do not resuscitate

LEARNING OUTCOMES

1. Define grief and loss.

2. What are Kubler-Ross's stages of grief?

3. List several common fears related to loss.

4. Describe three types of advance directives.

5. What is the difference between a do-not-resuscitate order and a comfort-measures-only order?

6. What is euthanasia?

7. List several manifestations of impending death.

8. Identify comfort measures for the client nearing death.

9. What is the role of hospice?

10. Describe the physiologic changes that indicate death.

APPLY WHAT YOU LEARNED

The nurse arrives to work at the hospice unit to find that there is a new admission. The client is a 84-year-old male with end-stage Alzheimer's disease. The client's daughter, son, and grandson are present for the admission. The client is unaware of his current surroundings and appears to be pleasant.

1. How would the nurse describe the type of care the client is going to receive to the family members?

2. How would the nurse explain nursing procedures to the client?

3. Explain the process of impending death as the nurse would explain to the family.

MULTIPLE CHOICE

Circle the answer that best completes the following statements.

1. A nursing student tells the nurse that she has heard the "death rattle" while caring for a client. The best explanation of this term is:
   A. creaking of the joints.
   B. gurgling of fluids in the lungs and throat.
   C. air bubbles in the stomach.
   D. teeth grinding.

2. Factors that may interfere with successful grieving include all of the following except:
   A. traumatic circumstances surrounding the loss.
   B. perceived inability to share the loss.
   C. lack of social recognition of the loss.
   D. mutual understanding and relationships.

3. The process of viewing the body after death best supports which of the following statements?
   A. Provides the resolution of the death experience for most families
   B. Increases anxiety levels
   C. Allows family members an avenue of escape from the truth
   D. Supports the family members' decision for a DNR

4. Which of the following would most likely interfere with the nurse–client relationship during the final stages of impending death?
   A. Unresolved issues of the nurse's perception of death
   B. Anger with the physician for writing a DNR order
   C. Inability to notify the client's family of the impending death
   D. Personal knowledge of the client's family situation

5. A nurse is caring for an elderly Chinese American and notices that a piece of handkerchief is lying on her chest. The nurse should immediately:
   A. throw the cloth in the trash.
   B. place the item on the bedside table.
   ✓C. speak to the family about the significance of the gesture.
   D. ignore the distraction.

6. An American Indian family appears to be throwing a party in the room where their grandmother is dying. Your best response would be to:
   A. remind the family of the seriousness of the situation.
   B. join in the festivities.
   ✓C. acknowledge the cultural tradition.
   D. report the incident to the nursing supervisor.

7. A nursing assistant refuses to care for a dying person. The most appropriate response by the nurse would be:
   A. "Okay, I'll reassign you to another patient."
   ✓B. "Please tell me what concerns you about this client's care."
   C. "Grow up, death is a part of life!"
   D. "Just get someone else to do this assignment for you."

8. Physical and emotional care is important to the dying person. Which of the following interventions would be the most comforting during the last stages of life?
   A. Change the linens every two hours.
   B. Provide frequent oral care.
   ✓C. Encourage a family member to spend time at the bedside.
   D. Tell the client that everything will be okay.

9. The concern that most clients voice as they near the end of their lives is:
   A. the fear of dying alone.
   ✓B. the fear of pain.
   C. the fear of leaving family members.
   D. the fear of bodily function loss.

10. You are helping another nurse to turn a comatose, dying client. The nurse states, "Whew, this lady sure is fat." Your best response should be:
    A. "That's not a nice thing to say."
    B. "Yeah, you got that right!"
    ✓C. "Let's talk outside after we are finished."
    D. Say nothing, just glare at the nurse.

11. A 94-year-old client refuses to eat breakfast. According to the shift report, she has not eaten in three days. Your next action should be to:
    A. keep trying to feed her by placing the food in her mouth.
    ✓B. read the physician's notes in her chart.
    C. call the family and ask them to bring food from home.
    D. start an IV of D$_5$W to provide calories.

12. Your client, diagnosed with inoperable stomach cancer, wants to die at home. He asks you what organization might help him die peacefully. Which of the following would be the most appropriate community referral resource?
   A. Meals-on-Wheels
   B. Community mental health centers
   ✓C. Hospice of America
   D. American Association of Colleges of Nursing

13. The nurse is aware that a terminal patient has stopped breathing, and responds to the call only after drinking a cup of coffee. This type of behavior is considered:
   A. routine in most facilities.
   ✓B. malpractice if the client has not been designated a DNR.
   C. unprofessional and inhumane.
   D. appropriate considering the client's prognosis.

14. You are caring for a client with end-stage renal disease. The client is fully alert and competent. The husband asks you to "give my wife just a little more pain medication to completely stop her from suffering." Your best response would be to:
   ✓A. clarify the request.
   B. privately administer more medication.
   C. speak to the wife about her pain level.
   D. call the physician and report the incident.

15. You overhear a client state, "If you make me well, God, I will try to be a better person." You know that this type of statement is one of the stages of the grieving process known as:
   A. anger.
   ✓B. bargaining.
   C. denial.
   D. depression.

Chapter 14

Caring for Clients Experiencing Shock, Trauma, or Disasters

EXPLORE PEARSON **mynursingkit**™

MyNursingKit is your one stop for online chapter review materials and resources. Prepare for success with additional NCLEX®-style practice questions, interactive assignments and activities, web links, animations and videos, and more!

Register your access code from the front of your book at
www.mynursingkit.com

KEY TERMS

Match each term with its appropriate definition.

H	1. Triage	A.	Discoloration of the skin
I	2. Shunt	B.	Diminished oxygenation to the tissues
J	3. Shock	C.	Irregular skin wound
G	4. Contusion	D.	Classification system used to determine illness level
D	5. Acuity	E.	Complete respiratory failure
E	6. ARDS	F.	Foreign substance
F	7. Antigen	G.	Injury to tissue without skin breakage
B	8. Hypoxia	H.	System to identify priority of care
A	9. Mottling	I.	Movement of fluids from one area to another
C	10. Laceration	J.	Life-threatening condition with inadequate blood flow to tissues and cells

LEARNING OUTCOMES

1. What is shock?

2. Name five types of shock.

3. Describe the three stages of shock.

4. What are manifestations of anaphylactic shock?

5. What is autotransfusion?

6. Identify the four types of blood and blood products.

7. List important nursing implications for blood transfusions.

8. What is trauma?

9. Contrast blunt and penetrating trauma.

10. Identify home safety tips to prevent injuries.

APPLY WHAT YOU LEARNED

A 22-year-old male enters the emergency department after being hit on the head with a baseball while watching a game. There is no active bleeding but he is complaining of a headache and some blurred vision. You notice that he is also holding his head where the injury occurred.

1. How would this injury be classified?

2. What assessment questions would the nurse ask in the triage department?

3. What diagnostic testing and treatments would the nurse expect to see ordered by the physician?

MULTIPLE CHOICE

Circle the answer that best completes the following statements.

1. Which of the following would not be considered the cause of a blood pressure drop in the condition known as shock?
   A. Loss of blood volume
   B. Severe histamine reaction
   C. Decreased cardiac output
   ✓D. Low HGB and HCT

2. A client with end-stage kidney disease is at risk for the progressive stage of shock because:
   A. the kidneys are not able to concentrate urine.
   ✓B. the renin-angiotensin system is not functioning properly.
   C. the kidneys are not able to metabolize toxins.
   D. the client is not at risk for this stage of shock.

3. Mr. Jones admits to the emergency room in shock after a motor vehicle crash. He is disoriented and unable to follow simple commands. You know that this is due to:
   ✓A. decreased blood flow to the brain.
   B. vasoconstriction of the great vessels.
   C. shunting of blood to the GI tract.
   D. the stress caused by the crash.

4. A person is most likely to experience an anaphylactic reaction:
   A. within five minutes of exposure to the allergen.
   B. after the second day of exposure to an allergen.
   C. when exposed to any allergen that produces hypersensitivity.
   ✓D. during the second exposure to the allergen.

5. Mrs. James is recovering from septic shock. She has extensive tissue damage to her liver and kidneys due to:
   A. bacterial infection.
   B. reaction to the antibiotic.
   ✓C. endotoxins released into the bloodstream.
   D. microemboli.

6. The administration of oxygen is an appropriate therapy for all types of shock because:
   A. oxygen eases the respiratory effort.
   ✓B. lack of oxygen is the primary cause of tissue damage.
   C. oxygen is considered a comforting measure.
   D. lack of oxygen increases the risk for mental confusion.

7. A client with B negative blood requires an emergency transfusion of whole blood. You know that in order to be compatible, the blood obtained from the lab must be:
   ✓A. O negative or B negative.
   B. O positive or B negative or B positive.
   C. B negative or AB negative.
   D. B positive or B negative.

8. The goal of epinephrine therapy is to:
   ✓A. promote bronchiole dilatation and increase arterial BP.
   B. reverse the histamine effects.
   C. prevent a delayed reaction to an antigen.
   D. prevent a delayed reaction to an antibody.

9. If there is blood loss or systemic vasodilation, you will expect the doctor to order:
   A. oxygen.
   ✓B. alpha-adrenergic medication.
   C. beta-adrenergic medication.
   D. cardiotonics.

10. Mr. Bruce has a nursing diagnosis of Ineffective Tissue Perfusion related to cardiopulmonary failure. Your primary nursing intervention will be to:
   ✓A. maintain airway and blood oxygen saturation.
   B. check vital signs every hour.
   C. obtain daily weights.
   D. assess bowel function every shift.

11. A client has been in the trauma room for 15 hours after experiencing a severe injury to her back. You suspect that the shock of the accident is resolving because:
   A. she stops asking where she is.
   ✓B. her urine output has increased to 40 mL/hr and the pedal pulses are palpable.
   C. oxygen saturation levels have been >94% for the last 60 minutes.
   D. her blood pressure is stable at 100/50.

12. You are pulled to the emergency room to assist with a sudden influx of patients. When you arrive, the charge nurse says to "pick a patient." Who will you see first?
   A. 50-year-old, chest pain, BP-140/80
   B. 26-year-old chronic asthmatic, R-30, O_2 saturation-92% room air, BP-120/72
   C. 18-year-old, leg trauma from a MVA, controlled hemorrhage, BP-139/80
   ✓D. 42-year-old, fall from roof, slurred speech, BP-80/40, P-160, R-36 shallow

13. The home health nurse is visiting 92-year-old Mr. Smith, who has been diagnosed with Parkinson's disease and early macular degeneration. Mr. Smith is at risk for trauma related to weakness and poor eyesight. Which of the following would decrease the fall potential for this client?
    A. Review the medications with the doctor.
    B. Assist the client in rearranging the furniture.
    C. Increase the number of lamps in the house.
    D. Encourage him to move into assisted-living housing.

14. Andrea has been diagnosed with an allergy to peanuts. You are providing nutritional education. You know that she needs further teaching when she says:
    A. "I need to ask what type of oil is used to fry the foods."
    B. "I need to read all food labels very carefully."
    C. "If I can't see the nuts, then I can eat the food."
    D. "I need to keep Benadryl with me at all times."

15. The school nurse is providing first-aid training to a group of high school athletic students. When she discusses hemorrhaging, she remembers to include:
    A. apply a tourniquet immediately to bleeding limbs.
    B. call for help, then apply a tourniquet.
    C. always move an injured person with the head lower than the feet.
    D. check for immediate danger, call for help, apply pressure.

Chapter 15

The Cardiovascular System and Assessment

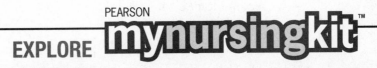

KEY TERMS

Match each term with its appropriate definition.

A 1. Sternum
E 2. Pericardium
F 3. Superior vena cava
I 4. Pulmonary artery
C 5. Coronary arteries
G 6. Sinoatrial node
J 7. Purkinje fibers
H 8. Depolarization
D 9. Internodal pathways
B 10. Tricuspid valve

A. Plate of bone forming the middle of the thorax

B. Flap of tissue between the right atrium and ventricle

C. Vessels that supply oxygen and nutrients to the cardiac muscle

D. Means for electrical currents to pass between nodes

E. Sac surrounding the heart and base of great vessels

F. Vessel that transports deoxygenated blood from upper body

G. Pacemaker of the heart

H. Reversal of positive and negative charges

I. Vessel that carries deoxygenated blood from the right ventricle

J. The last part of the heart conduction system

LEARNING OUTCOMES

1. Describe the heart.

2. Contrast diastole and systole.
   Rest and contract

3. What is the peripheral vascular system?
   Extremities

4. Describe an ECG.

5. What is contractility?
   When the heart contracts

6. Explain cardiac output.
   HR x SV

7. List several components that affect heart rate.

8. Identify components of a lipid profile.

9. What imaging studies are used in cardiac dysfunction?
   EKG echocardiogram

10. What is the purpose of a cardiac MRI?
    Take a 3D picture of the heart

APPLY WHAT YOU LEARNED

A nursing student is learning the disruptions related to the cardiac system. The student knows that a complete physical examination is important in order to provide proper treatment to the client. The student also knows that assessments need to be performed in a timely manner, especially in acute situations.

1. Describe the type of assessment to be done on a client experiencing chest pain.

2. Identify diagnostic testing in cardiac dysfunction.

MULTIPLE CHOICE

Circle the answer that best completes the following statements.

1. The AV valves close as the ventricles start to contract, producing the first heart sound called:
   - A. S_1.
   - B. S_2.
   - C. S_3.
   - D. S_4.

2. The heartbeat is controlled by specialized cells within the myocardium known as the:
   - A. nervous system.
   - B. respiratory system.
   - C. conduction system.
   - D. cardiac system.

3. The sinoatrial (SA) node usually generates an impulse:
   - A. 40 to 60 times per minute.
   - B. 50 times per minute.
   - C. 60 to 100 times per minute.
   - D. 100 times per minute.

4. The action potential and depolarization cause muscle to:
   - A. beat.
   - B. contract.
   - C. twitch.
   - D. elevate.

5. Ventricular filling occurs when the ventricles are relaxed during:
   - A. systole.
   - B. heartbeat.
   - C. contraction.
   - D. diastole.

6. Arteries, veins, and capillaries are included in the:
   - A. cardiac system.
   - B. GI system.
   - C. peripheral vascular system.
   - D. pulmonary system.

7. A noninvasive test that has been shown to be highly indicative of atherosclerosis is called a(n):
   - A. ankle-brachial index.
   - B. ECG.
   - C. femoral-cephalic index.
   - D. Holter monitor.

8. These hormones are released by the heart muscle in response to changes in blood volume:
   A. ANF.
   B. estrogen.
   C. BMP.
   D. testosterone.

9. Stress testing is used to detect asymptomatic coronary heart disease and may cause:
   A. an increase in pulse rate.
   B. exhaustion.
   C. an increase in stress.
   D. a cardiac emergency.

10. A transthoracic echocardiogram (TTE) is:
    A. expensive.
    B. dangerous.
    C. invasive.
    D. noninvasive.

11. Which part of the heart receives deoxygenated blood from the veins of the body?
    A. Left atrium
    B. Right atrium
    C. Left ventricle
    D. Right ventricle

12. Which structure is known as the "pacemaker" of the heart?
    A. Sinoatrial node
    B. Bundle of His
    C. Purkinje fibers
    D. Left bundle branch

13. The force that opposes blood flow is known as:
    A. arterial resistance.
    B. peripheral vascular resistance.
    C. ventricular resistance.
    D. regurgitation.

14. Which of the following is not a part of a lipid profile?
    A. BNP
    B. HDL
    C. LDL
    D. VLDL

15. The bicuspid valve is also known as the:
    A. pulmonary valve.
    B. mitral valve.
    C. aortic valve.
    D. tricuspid valve.

Chapter 16

Caring for Clients With Coronary Heart Disease and Dysrhythmias

KEY TERMS

Match each term with its appropriate definition.

C 1. CAD   A. Profuse sweating

G 2. Atherosclerosis   B. An amino acid linked to CAD

I 3. Angina pectoris   C. Impaired blood flow to the heart muscle

A 4. Diaphoresis   D. Muscle aches

E 5. Metabolic syndrome   E. A group of related risk factors for coronary heart disease

B 6. Homocysteine   F. Without enough blood and oxygen to meet metabolic needs

F 7. Ischemic   G. A narrowing of the coronary arteries due to plaque formation

D 8. Myalgias   H. Impaired tissue perfusion due to pump failure

J 9. Prinzmetal's   I. Episodic chest pain

H 10. Cardiogenic shock   J. Atypical angina that occurs without an identified precipitating cause, often waking the client from sleep

LEARNING OUTCOMES

1. List several risk factors for coronary heart disease.

2. What is atherosclerosis?

3. Describe manifestations of angina.

4. List several manifestations of an acute myocardial infarction.

5. What are cardiac dysrhythmias?

6. What is cardioversion?

7. Define sudden cardiac death.

8. List medications in the class known as calcium channel blockers.

9. What are premature ventricular contractions?

10. Define atrial flutter.

APPLY WHAT YOU LEARNED

You are admitting a client for a pacemaker insertion. The client tells you that they have not eaten anything past midnight and have not smoked any cigarettes in the past 24 hours. The client's wife and teenage daughter are present and will be providing care for him at home.

1. Identify teaching for the client and the family.

2. What are nursing diagnoses related to this client?

3. When should the client call his physician?

MULTIPLE CHOICE

Circle the answer that best completes the following statements.

1. The nurse is explaining the purpose of an electrocardiogram to a group of nursing students. The nurse would be correct if she said:
   A. "It allows the doctor to view the inside of the heart."
   B. "It produces a picture of the electrical activity of the heart."
   C. "It is used to increase the diameter of the artery."
   D. "It is a device that temporarily takes over the function of the SA node."

2. If all of the following are true, which assessment data should be the highest priority for the nurse to obtain from the client with a dysrhythmia?
   A. History of falls
   B. Smoking habits
   C. History of cardiovascular disease
   D. Current medications

3. A client has received instructions on his new pacemaker. Which of these comments, if made by the client, indicates a need for further teaching?
   A. "I'll carry my pacemaker card in my wallet."
   B. "If my pulse drops lower than the set rate, I'll take a rest break."
   C. "I will call the doctor if I have any chest pain."
   D. "I should see my doctor on a regular schedule."

4. You are walking in the parking lot at the grocery store when you see a woman lying by her car. Your next action should be:
   A. call for help.
   B. begin CPR.
   C. ask the woman if she is okay.
   D. check for a pulse.

5. A client presents to the clinic with complaints of orthopnea and severe pedal edema. He tells the nurse that he is taking Lasix and digoxin for congestive heart failure. The assessment reveals an elevated BP, crackles throughout the lung fields and 3+ pitting edema. The most appropriate nursing diagnosis would be:
    A. Noncompliance.
    B. Ineffective Cardiac Tissue Perfusion.
    C. Risk for Skin Impairment.
    D. Excess Fluid Volume.

6. Several hours after a client has returned from a coronary angiography, you notice that the dressing is saturated with blood. Your next action should be to:
    A. call the doctor.
    B. check for a pulse distal to the incision.
    C. reinforce the dressing.
    D. apply pressure to the site.

7. Which of the following would not be discussed with a client scheduled for cardiac surgery?
    A. Coughing and deep breathing exercises
    B. Special cardiac diet prior to the surgery
    C. Visiting hours after the surgery
    D. Proper use of antiembolic hose

8. A client asks you if his cholesterol level of 210 is within the normal range. Your response should be:
    A. "It all depends on which level you are talking about, the total or the LDL."
    B. "That is high. It should be under 200."
    C. "You have to ask your doctor about that."
    D. "I'm not sure. Let me go check my lab reference book."

9. A client is to receive a morning dose of digoxin. Which finding, if present, would indicate that the medication should not be given?
    A. Radial pulse of 80
    B. Apical pulse of 52
    C. Radial pulse of 60
    D. Apical pulse of 62

10. A client with a history of rheumatic heart disease has been scheduled for a tooth extraction. Which of the following would the nurse anticipate the dentist will prescribe for this client before the procedure?
    A. Anticoagulant
    B. Antibiotic
    C. Cardiotonic
    D. ACE inhibitor

11. Which of the following drugs is a beta blocker?
    A. Procan
    B. Quinidine
    C. Inderal
    D. Cardizem

12. Which drug class can also cause dysrhythmias?
    A. Beta blockers
    B. Calcium channel blockers
    C. Digoxins
    D. All of the above

13. What is the first step in the CPR sequence?
    A. Call for help
    B. Assess for responsiveness
    C. Open the airway with head tilt-chin lift
    D. Provide two rescue breaths

14. Death will follow the onset of V-fib if not treated in:
    A. 30 seconds
    B. 4 minutes
    C. 2 minutes
    D. 10 minutes

15. Nitroglycerin tablets are given via which method?
    A. Topical
    B. Transdermal
    C. Sublingual
    D. Rectal

Chapter 17

Caring for Clients With Cardiac Disorders

EXPLORE **mynursingkit**
PEARSON

MyNursingKit is your one stop for online chapter review materials and resources. Prepare for success with additional NCLEX®-style practice questions, interactive assignments and activities, web links, animations and videos, and more!

Register your access code from the front of your book at
www.mynursingkit.com

KEY TERMS

Match each term with its appropriate definition.

_I_	1.	Heart failure	A. Wrapping a skeletal muscle graft around the heart to lend support to the failing myocardium
_E_	2.	Ventricular hypertrophy	B. Breathing difficulty while lying down
_G_	3.	Cardiac reserve	C. Condition in which the client awakens at night acutely short of breath
_B_	4.	Orthopnea	D. Inflammation of the endocardium, an infectious process that usually affects clients with underlying heart disease
_J_	5.	Pulmonary edema	E. Enlarged cardiac muscle cells
_C_	6.	PND	F. Drug that increases the strength of the heart's contractions
_E_	7.	Inotropic	G. Ability of the heart to adjust its output to meet the metabolic needs of the body
_A_	8.	Cardiomyoplasty	H. A systemic inflammatory disease caused by an abnormal immune response to infection by group A beta-hemolytic streptococci
_H_	9.	Rheumatic fever	I. The inability of the heart to function as a pump to meet the needs of the body
_D_	10.	Endocarditis	J. Accumulation of fluid in the interstitial spaces and alveoli of the lungs

LEARNING OUTCOMES

1. What is heart failure?

2. Identify teaching points for older adults regarding changes in cardiovascular function.

3. What are the classifications for heart failure?

4. What is rheumatic fever?

5. List several manifestations of rheumatic fever.

6. What are the indications for prophylactic antibiotics to prevent endocarditis?

7. Define pericarditis.

8. Identify types of heart murmurs.

9. What is cardiomyopathy?

10. Describe mitral valve prolapse.

APPLY WHAT YOU LEARNED

Your client was admitted through the ER and is to have valvuloplasty in the morning. He has no family present and did not provide you with any contact information of any other relatives. He states that he lives alone in a two-story home and has to climb 15 stairs to get to his bedroom.

1. What nursing care would be applied to this client after surgery?

2. What other disciplines would the nurse involve in the treatment of this client?

3. What education should the nurse provide about activity intolerance?

MULTIPLE CHOICE

Circle the answer that best completes the following statements.

1. You are instructing a nursing student in the correct administration of a nitro-glycerin patch. The most important point that should be made at this time is to:
   A. wipe off the old medication before applying the new patch.
   B. rotate sites.
   C. wear gloves.
   D. not massage into the skin.

2. A client has been admitted to the hospital in acute heart failure. Which of the following diets would the nurse expect to see ordered for the patient?
   A. Low-fat, high-protein
   B. High-potassium, low-protein
   C. Low-sodium, high-protein
   D. High-protein, high-sodium

3. Which of the following nursing diagnoses would be most appropriate for the client in congestive heart failure?
   A. Activity Intolerance
   B. Deficient Knowledge
   C. Pain, Acute
   D. Deficient Fluid Volume

4. A client in end-stage renal disease has been diagnosed with pericarditis. Which intervention would the nurse expect to include in the nursing care plan?
   A. Assist with a pericardiocentesis
   B. Administer NSAIDs
   C. Assess the lung sounds every eight hours
   D. Place the bed in low-Fowler's position

5. A 28-year-old female, pregnant with her second child, arrives in the emergency room with severe SOB and hemoptysis. The physician tells you that the client's lungs are "wet" and that he is able to detect a diastolic murmur. You suspect that this client has:
   A. aspiration pneumonia.
   B. pulmonary edema.
   C. right-sided heart failure.
   D. cardiac tamponade.

6. Valvular heart disease interferes with blood flow to and from the heart. The most common cause of this disease is:
   A. pericarditis.
   B. MI.
   C. CHF.
   D. rheumatic fever.

7. Valve disorders affect pressures and blood flow both in front of and behind the affected valve. The two major types of heart valve disorders are:
   A. aspiration and pneumonia.
   B. pulmonic and edema.
   C. stenosis and regurgitation.
   D. cardiac and pulmonic.

8. A 34-year-old female, pregnant with her first child, arrives in the emergency room with severe SOB, fatigue, and palpitations. The physician tells you that he is able to detect a diastolic murmur. You suspect that this client has:
   A. mitral regurgitation.
   B. mitral stenosis.
   C. right-sided heart failure.
   D. cardiac tamponade.

9. You are assessing your client and hear a "seagull-like" murmur at the apex of his heart. You suspect that this client has:
   A. mitral regurgitation.
   B. mitral stenosis.
   C. right-sided heart failure.
   D. cardiac tamponade.

10. A 56-year-old client presents with angina, dyspnea, and syncope. His prognosis is grim; most clients get progressively worse and die within two years of the onset of symptoms. You suspect that this client has:
    A. cardiac tamponade.
    B. myocarditis.
    C. cardiomyopathy.
    D. pericarditis.

11. The most common cause of right ventricular failure is:
    A. left ventricular failure.
    B. right atrial failure.
    C. left atrial failure.
    D. pulmonary failure.

12. The drug class that increases the strength of the heart's contractions is known as:
    A. calcium channel blockers.
    B. inotropics.
    C. analgesics.
    D. beta blockers.

13. A common side effect of an ACE inhibitor is:
    A. runny nose.
    B. cough.
    C. nausea.
    D. tinnitus.

14. Cardiac clients need to weigh themselves daily. They should know that 1 kg is equal to:
    A. 2.2 kg.
    B. 5 lbs.
    C. 2.2 lbs.
    D. 2.2 cm.

15. Rheumatic fever is usually caused by:
    A. staphylococcus.
    B. streptococcus.
    C. clostridium.
    D. E. coli.

Chapter 18

Caring for Clients With Peripheral Vascular Disorders

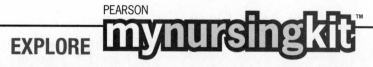

EXPLORE PEARSON **mynursingkit**™

MyNursingKit is your one stop for online chapter review materials and resources. Prepare for success with additional NCLEX®-style practice questions, interactive assignments and activities, web links, animations and videos, and more!

Register your access code from the front of your book at
www.mynursingkit.com

KEY TERMS

Match each term with its appropriate definition.

E   1. Capillary   A.   Inner layer of vessel wall

F   2. Tunica adventitia   B.   Special cells that are sensitive to chemicals

D   3. Valves   C.   Middle layer of vessel containing smooth muscle

C   4. Tunica media   D.   Located in vessels to prevent backflow of blood

A   5. Tunica intima   E.   Minute vessel that connects arterioles and venules

I   6. Arterioles   F.   Protects and anchors vessels

H   7. Baroreceptors   G.   Thickness of a substance

G   8. Viscosity   H.   Cells that are sensitive to blood pressure changes

J   9. PVR   I.   Tiny arterial branch

B   10. Chemoreceptors   J.   Opposing forces to blood flow

LEARNING OUTCOMES

1. Define hypertension.

2. Identify risk factors for hypertension.

3. Describe manifestations of an abdominal aortic aneurysm.

4. Define Marfan syndrome.

5. Describe arteriosclerosis.

6. Identify complementary therapies in peripheral vascular disease (PVD).

7. Define Raynaud's phenomenon.

8. Identify risk factors for venous thrombosis.

9. Define varicose veins.

10. Describe manifestations of varicose veins.

APPLY WHAT YOU LEARNED

A 22-year-old women presents to the ER with complaints of stiffness and decreased sensation in her hands. Upon inspection, you notice that her hands change from blue to white in color. The client tells you that her fingers usually turn red after the blueness goes away.

1. What would the nurse suspect the diagnosis to be in this client?

2. Identify treatments regarding this client.

MULTIPLE CHOICE

Circle the answer that best completes the following statements.

1. Mr. Greggs, age 68, is being seen in the clinic for a routine physical. He is of Jewish ancestry. He tells you that he smokes a half-pack of cigarettes per day and enjoys popcorn and sodas as a snack. His weight is 205 pounds. Which of these risk factors is considered unalterable in the prevention of hypertension?
   A. Family history
   B. Smoking
   C. High sodium intake
   D. Obesity

2. The nurse is teaching the assistant how to take a blood pressure. Further teaching is indicated if the assistant:
   A. centers the cuff directly over the artery.
   B. palpates the artery before beginning the procedure.
   C. inflates the cuff 80 mm Hg over the pulse level.
   D. closes the cuff at 40% arm circumference.

3. Which of the following should be included on a nursing care plan for a client with peripheral vascular disease?
   A. Dry the feet carefully by rubbing briskly.
   B. Buy shoes in the morning before swelling begins.
   C. Check the temperature of the water before stepping into the tub.
   D. Do not use powder on the feet.

4. You are caring for a client who has had aortic surgery. You know to assess for signs of graft leakage. If all of the following are true, which would be considered the highest priority for nursing intervention?
   A. Hematoma at the incision
   B. Decreasing peripheral pulses
   C. Increased abdominal girth
   D. Decreasing blood pressure

5. The nurse is preparing a care plan for a client with DVT. All of the following nursing diagnoses are appropriate except:
   A. Pain, Acute
   B. Ineffective Peripheral Tissue Perfusion
   C. Impaired Skin Integrity
   D. Risk for Constipation

6. A client, diagnosed with HTN, has been started on an ACE inhibitor. You know that the action of this medication to reduce blood pressure is due to:
   A. blocking the sympathetic input to the heart.
   B. inhibition of the renin–angiotensin–aldosterone mechanism.
   C. slowing the heart rate by reducing vasoconstriction.
   D. relaxation of vascular smooth muscle.

7. Your client has a blood pressure of 164/100. You anticipate that the physician will:
   A. recheck the BP in one year.
   B. confirm the BP within two months.
   C. refer for evaluation within one month.
   D. refer for evaluation within one week.

8. You are teaching a client about a diet low in vitamin K. You know that the client understands the instructions because she tells you that:
   A. "I will buy boxed macaroni and cheese instead of making it from scratch."
   B. "I will eat lots of yogurt because I need the calcium."
   C. "I will buy 1% milk from now on."
   D. "I will stop buying spinach for a few months."

9. A 46-year-old executive asks you to help him understand how to reduce the stress in his life. He has recently been diagnosed with primary hypertension. Your best response should be:
   A. "Stop worrying about everything."
   B. "Exercise regularly everyday."
   C. "Take a class that focuses on therapeutic touch."
   D. "Join a meditation group."

10. The primary manifestation of peripheral arterial disease is:
    A. pain.
    B. dependent rubor.
    C. intermittent claudication.
    D. decreased pulses.

11. A client with DVT suddenly develops chest pain and SOB. The nurse suspects that this client has developed:
    A. an embolism.
    B. atelectasis.
    C. spontaneous pneumothorax.
    D. bacterial pneumonia.

12. During the physical assessment, the nurse discovers that there are no palpable pedal pulses in the client's left foot. Her next action should be to:
    A. reattempt to palpate the pulses.
    B. ask the charge nurse to palpate the pulses.
    C. obtain a Doppler.
    D. document the absent pulses.

13. A client has been diagnosed with severe peripheral vascular disease. The nurse anticipates that the physician will order a low dose of aspirin. The rationale for the use of this medication is that:
    A. aspirin decreases the risk for clot formation.
    B. aspirin is an analgesic.
    C. aspirin can prevent a fever from occurring.
    D. aspirin is contraindicated in the client with PVD.

14. You are discussing nursing interventions with the charge nurse for a client with PVD. You suggest that the following intervention should be included:
    A. Gatch the knee at a 90-degree angle.
    B. Instruct the client to keep the extremity in an independent position.
    C. Use a heating pad to keep the extremity warm.
    D. Assess the peripheral pulses every four hours.

15. The physician has prescribed the drug Coumadin for a client with arterial disease. Which of the following should be included in the client teaching?
    A. Increase the amount of vitamin K in the diet.
    B. Report any unusual bruises.
    C. Have blood levels of the medication taken every six months.
    D. Double the dose of the medication if a dose is skipped.

Chapter 19

The Hematologic and Lymphatic Systems and Assessment

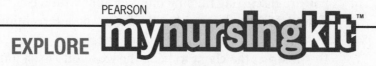

KEY TERMS

Match each term with its appropriate definition.

✓ C	1. Plasma	A.	An essential part of the body's clotting mechanism
✓ F	2. Stem cells	B.	Hormone that stimulates the bone marrow to produce RBCs
✓ G	3. Erythrocytes	C.	A clear yellow, protein-rich fluid
✓ B	4. Erythropoietin	D.	An oxygen-carrying protein
D	5. Hemoglobin	E.	Part of the body's defense against infection and disease
✓ J	6. Hemolysis	F.	The beginning of all cells
H	7. Transferrin	G.	Shaped like *biconcave disks*
✓ E	8. Leukocytes	H.	Iron that circulates in the bloodstream
✓ I	9. Phagocytes	I.	Responsible for engulfing and destroying foreign matter
✓ A	10. Platelets	J.	The process of RBC destruction

LEARNING OUTCOMES

1. Define plasma.

2. Describe hemoglobin.

3. Identify differential components in WBCs.

4. Define platelets.

5. Describe the lymphatic system.

6. Identify lab tests used in lymphatic disorders.

7. Describe a bone marrow aspiration.

8. Identify the five stages in hemostasis.

9. Discuss the purpose of blood.

10. Identify the normal hemoglobin count in men and women.

APPLY WHAT YOU LEARNED

A 38-year-old woman presents to the physician's office with complaints of fatigue, easy bruising, and a bruise on her leg that she states has been there for at least a month. Upon further assessment, she tells you that she sleeps as much as possible and cannot tolerate much activity. Her appetite is poor and she is currently not taking any medications.

1. What diagnostic testing would the nurse expect with this client?

2. What teaching would the nurse provide to the client regarding some of the diagnostic testing?

MULTIPLE CHOICE

Circle the answer that best completes the following statements.

1. A laboratory test used to diagnose hemolytic anemias and investigate transfusion reactions is called:
   A. electrophoresis.
   B. coagulation.
   C. Coombs'.
   D. Schilling's.

2. Before a bone marrow aspiration, the nurse should have the client:
   A. maintain a full bladder.
   B. lie in reverse Trendelenburg position.
   C. sign an informed consent.
   D. cough.

3. A client is undergoing a biopsy to rule out malignancy of her left supraclavicular lymph node. The nurse tells her prior to the procedure:
   A. "You can't eat for 24 hours after the procedure."
   B. "You will bleed excessively following the procedure."
   C. "You are only allowed two visitors every thirty minutes."
   D. "I will monitor your vital signs routinely after the procedure."

4. The primary function of RBCs is to:
   A. transport oxygen to the cells.
   B. provide immunity to the body.
   C. destroy foreign matter.
   D. control bleeding.

5. Mr. Kelp is diagnosed with iron-deficiency anemia. You should recommend a diet of increased:
   A. organ meats.
   B. fruits.
   C. bread.
   D. dairy products.

6. A Schilling test is used to diagnose:
   A. addiction.
   B. pernicious anemia.
   C. aplastic anemia.
   D. cancer.

7. Mary, 11, was diagnosed with leukemia. The nurse knows to watch for what observation in her assessment?
   A. Scales and rashes
   B. Petechiae and purpura
   C. Bowel and bladder control
   D. Loss of sensation

8. The most serious hazard for a client who has had a bone marrow aspiration is:
   A. hemorrhage.
   B. pain.
   C. bruising.
   D. shock.

9. This evaluates the extrinsic clotting pathway, which is prolonged in Coumadin therapy:
   A. INR
   B. PTT
   C. PT
   D. APTT

10. A 28-year-old client's transferrin lab has come back slightly elevated. You ask her if she is taking:
    A. cocaine.
    B. amphetamines.
    C. Coumadin.
    D. oral contraceptives.

11. Normal hemoglobin for a woman should be in the range of:
    A. 12–15 g/dL
    B. 5–10 g/dL
    C. 15–20 g/dL
    D. 30–35 g/dL

12. RBCs have a life span of about:
    A. 30 days.
    B. 120 days.
    C. 45 days.
    D. 90 days.

13. WBCs are also called:
    A. platelets.
    B. erythrocytes.
    C. leukocytes.
    D. phagocytes.

14. The most plentiful of the WBCs are:
    A. granulocytes.
    B. eosinophils.
    C. basophils.
    D. monocytes.

15. What term is used to describe blood clotting?
    A. Hemostasis
    B. Hemocytoblastosis
    C. Erythrocytosis
    D. Homeostasis

Chapter 20

Caring for Clients With Hematologic and Lymphatic Disorders

KEY TERMS

Match each term with its appropriate definition.

___C___ 1. Anemia

___H___ 2. Polycythemia

___I___ 3. Myeloma

___B___ 4. Leukemia

___G___ 5. Agranulocytosis

___D___ 6. Hemophilia

___A___ 7. DIC

___J___ 8. Lymphangitis

___F___ 9. Malignant lymphoma

___E___ 10. Thrombocytopenia

A. A complex disorder characterized by simultaneous blood clotting and hemorrhages

B. A group of malignant disorders of WBCs

C. Hemoglobin concentration, or the number of circulating RBCs, is decreased

D. A group of hereditary clotting factor deficiencies

E. A platelet count of less than 100,000 platelets per milliliter of blood

F. Condition characterized by lymphocyte proliferation

G. A decrease in granulocytes

H. Excess erythropoietin production

I. Malignancy in which plasma cells multiply uncontrollably and infiltrate bone marrow, lymph nodes, and other tissues

J. Inflammation of the lymph vessels

LEARNING OUTCOMES

1. Define anemia.

2. Describe thalassemia.

3. Identify dietary sources of folic acid.

4. Define polycythemia.

5. Describe manifestations of leukemia.

6. Identify the four major classifications of leukemia.

7. Identify nursing diagnoses involved with leukemia.

8. Define agranulocytosis.

9. Describe thrombocytopenia.

10. Identify risk factors for disseminated intravascular coagulation.

APPLY WHAT YOU LEARNED

Upon assessment of a new client on your wing, you discover enlarged lymph nodes and a fever. When talking to the client, you find out that the client has been having night sweats, fatigue, and weight loss. They also complain about itchy skin and malaise. The client tells you that this has been going on for a few weeks.

1. What would the manifestations above mean in terms of diagnosis?

2. What treatment options are available for this client?

3. What nursing diagnoses apply to this situation?

MULTIPLE CHOICE

Circle the answer that best completes the following statements.

1. Acquired hemolytic anemia results when RBCs are damaged by outside factors, such as:
   A. immune responses.
   B. cellular development.
   C. healing.
   D. stress.

2. Aplastic anemia may follow injury to stem cells in bone marrow caused by:
   A. certain infections.
   B. drugs or radiation.
   C. chemicals.
   D. all of the above.

3. Aplastic anemia, if left untreated, could ultimately lead to:
   A. leukocytosis.
   B. leukopenia.
   C. nothing; it corrects itself.
   D. heart failure.

4. Sickle cell anemia usually affects people of:
   A. Mediterranean descent.
   B. Asian descent.
   C. African descent.
   D. European descent.

5. Myelodysplastic syndrome (MDS) is a group of stem cell disorders characterized by abnormal-appearing bone marrow and ineffective blood cell production. It is primarily a disorder of:
   A. middle adults.
   B. young adults.
   C. older adults.
   D. children.

6. After an autologous bone marrow transplant, the risk of death is greater for a client due to:
   A. microorganisms.
   B. bleeding.
   C. immunosuppression.
   D. pain.

7. An alternative to bone marrow transplant is:
   A. brain cell transplant.
   B. stem cell transplant.
   C. spinal fluid transplant.
   D. all of the above.

8. The inheritance patterns for both hemophilia A and B are:
   A. Y-linked recessive disorders.
   B. X-linked recessive disorders.
   C. female reproductive disorders.
   D. male reproductive disorders.

9. A person with Hodgkin's may have a nursing diagnosis of:
   A. Risk for Impaired Skin Integrity.
   B. Disturbed Thought Processes.
   C. Deficient Fluid Volume.
   D. None of the above.

10. Exposure to environmental toxins such as radiation and benzene, and cancer treatment with radiation and chemotherapy, are identified risk factors for:
    A. AIDS.
    B. BMT.
    C. SCT.
    D. MDS.

11. A condition where the concentration of hemoglobin is decreased is known as:
    A. anemia.
    B. amenorrhea.
    C. anorexia.
    D. agranulocytosis.

12. People receiving TPN may develop a deficiency in:
    A. glucose.
    B. chloride.
    C. folate.
    D. lipids.

13. Thalassemia usually affects which group?
    A. African Americans
    B. Caucasians
    C. Mediterranean
    D. Canadians

14. Dietary sources of iron include all of the following except:
    A. beef.
    B. pork.
    C. cheese.
    D. potatoes.

15. An excessively high red blood cell count is known as:
    A. polycythemia.
    B. leukemia.
    C. anemia.
    D. thalassemia.

Chapter 21

The Respiratory System and Assessment

KEY TERMS

Match each term with its appropriate definition.

B	1. Vocal cords	A.	Located between laryngopharynx and trachea
I	2. Eustachian tubes	B.	Mucous membranes that produce speech
H	3. Nares	C.	Filter air as it enters the nose
D	4. Nasopharynx	D.	Contains the tonsils and adenoids
J	5. Epiglottis	E.	Trap large particles within nasal cavity
A	6. Larynx	F.	Openings in facial bones that lighten the skull
E	7. Turbinates	G.	Prevents food from entering nasopharynx
F	8. Sinuses	H.	External opening of nasal cavity
C	9. Nasal hairs	I.	Connects middle ear and nasopharynx
G	10. Soft palate	J.	Closes during swallowing to prevent aspiration

LEARNING OUTCOMES

1. Describe the function of the upper respiratory system.

2. Identify structures of the upper respiratory system.

3. Describe the function of the lower respiratory system.

4. Identify structures of the lower respiratory system.

5. Discuss respiratory changes associated with aging.

6. Define adventitious breath sounds.

7. Describe pulse oximetry.

8. Describe the procedure to obtain a throat swab.

9. Identify the purpose of the ventilation-perfusion scan.

10. Discuss client and family teaching regarding bronchoscopy procedures.

APPLY WHAT YOU LEARNED

A 72-year-old male presents to the clinic with complaints of "flu-like symptoms." He tells you that he has had a sore throat for the past four days with a dry, nonproductive cough. The client denies allergies and chronic illness.

1. Describe the nursing assessment that will be performed for this client.

2. What diagnostic testing would the nurse expect to see ordered by the physician?

3. What other pertinent data would the nurse ask the client in reference to the "flu-like symptoms"?

MULTIPLE CHOICE

Circle the answer that best completes the following statements.

1. The primary laboratory tests used to evaluate the respiratory system and diagnose disorders affecting it are:
   A. tissue biopsy, pulse oximetry, and arterial blood gases.
   B. arterial blood gases, tissue biopsy, and nasal, throat, and sputum cultures.
   C. nasal, throat, and sputum cultures, ear swab, tissue biopsy.
   D. tissue biopsy, arterial blood gases, and blood glucose.

2. Tissue for biopsy, or microscopic examination, may be obtained by needle aspiration of a:
   A. lymph node.
   B. brain cell.
   C. spinal membrane.
   D. bronchus.

3. Lung volume and capacity are measured with:
   A. LCDs.
   B. PETs.
   C. LATs.
   D. PFTs.

4. You are teaching a client going for a pulmonary function test to stop using bronchodilators, drinking caffeinated beverages, or smoking 4–6 hours before the test because:
   A. they could die.
   B. testing policy dictates.
   C. bronchodilators, smoking, and caffeine interfere with test results.
   D. the results will always be positive.

5. Marta, age 25, has asthma. She uses a peak expiratory flow rate (PEFR) meter on a day-to-day basis to:
   A. monitor air humidity.
   B. assess her breathing pattern.
   C. monitor airway constriction.
   D. balance the amount of rest periods and activities.

6. Jason, age 38, was diagnosed with laryngeal tumors via:
   A. laryngoscopy.
   B. bronchoscopy.
   C. EGD.
   D. EEG.

7. A patent airway and unobstructed airflow are vital to sustain life and:
   A. well-being.
   B. lung capacity.
   C. function.
   D. love.

8. Before doing a CT of the head and neck, an important nursing implication is to inquire about:
   A. consent.
   B. next of kin.
   C. bleeding.
   D. allergies.

9. Following arterial puncture, the nurse often is responsible for applying pressure to the site for a period of:
   A. 5 to 10 minutes.
   B. 30 minutes.
   C. 2 to 5 minutes.
   D. 1 hour.

10. A detergent-like substance that helps keep alveoli open is called:
    A. mainstem.
    B. hilus.
    C. surfactant.
    D. bronchus.

11. During inspiration, the diaphragm:
    A. contracts and flattens out.
    B. dilates and fills out.
    C. constricts and releases gases.
    D. holds on to air.

12. In a client with barrel chest, the chest is:
    A. decreased in anterior-posterior diameter.
    B. increased in anterior-posterior diameter.
    C. symmetrical in diameter.
    D. concave in diameter.

13. The pharynx is a passageway for:
    A. food.
    B. bile.
    C. singing.
    D. bronchi.

14. The nasopharynx starts at the:
    A. mouth.
    B. tongue.
    C. nose.
    D. throat.

15. The double-layered membrane that covers the lungs is called:
    A. pleura.
    B. bronchi.
    C. rales.
    D. trachea.

Chapter 22

Caring for Clients With Upper Respiratory Disorders

KEY TERMS

Match each term with its appropriate definition.

D 1. Rhinitis
B 2. Influenza
E 3. Sinusitis
I 4. Pharyngitis
F 5. Tonsillitis
A 6. Otalgia
G 7. Stridor
C 8. Aphonia
H 9. Echinacea
J 10. Dyspnea

A. Pain in the ear

B. A highly contagious viral respiratory disease

C. Complete loss of the voice

D. Inflammation of the nasal cavities

E. Inflammation of the mucous membranes of the sinuses

F. Acute inflammation of the tonsils

G. A high-pitched, harsh sound heard during inspiration

H. Herbal remedy that may reduce the duration and symptoms of a common cold or influenza

I. Acute inflammation of the throat

J. Difficult or labored breathing

LEARNING OUTCOMES

1. Identify manifestations of acute pharyngitis.

2. Define rhinitis and sinusitis.

3. Describe people who should receive annual influenza vaccines.

4. Describe methods of nursing care in controlling URIs in long-term care.

5. Define stridor.

6. Identify some nursing diagnoses of clients with URIs.

7. Describe pertussis.

8. Define epistaxis.

9. Identify manifestations of nasal fractures.

10. Describe sleep apnea.

APPLY WHAT YOU LEARNED

A 61-year-old man presents to the clinic for follow-up regarding his diagnosis of laryngeal cancer. He continues to smoke 2 ppd and drinks 3–4 alcoholic drinks per day. His voice is hoarse and offers complaints of a sore throat and decreased appetite. Total laryngectomy is suggested at this time by the physician.

1. How would the nurse explain the importance of abstaining from alcohol (ETOH) and cigarettes?

2. Describe teaching regarding a total laryngectomy.

3. Discuss postoperative care for this client.

MULTIPLE CHOICE

Circle the answer that best completes the following statements.

1. Before administering the polyvalent influenza virus vaccine to a patient, the nurse should:
   A. ask the patient about previous flu episodes.
   B. obtain vital signs.
   C. note patient allergies to eggs.
   D. request the patient to sign an informed consent.

2. The client who is receiving antibiotics for a bacterial infection is no longer contagious after:
   A. 12 hours.
   B. 24 hours.
   C. 48 hours.
   D. 72 hours.

3. Which of the following medications, if used longer than 3 to 5 days, may result in rebound congestion?
   A. Fexofenadine
   B. Neo-Synephrine
   C. Clesmastine
   D. Allegra

4. You are assigned to assist in writing the discharge plans for a client who has had endoscopic sinus surgery. Client teaching should include:
   A. sneeze into a tissue to prevent spreading of microorganisms.
   B. no lifting restrictions for three days.
   C. avoid smoking.
   D. notify the physician for a temperature greater than 100°F.

5. Nursing interventions for the diagnosis of Ineffective Airway Clearance should include:
   A. balance the amount of rest periods and activities.
   B. assess the client's sleep patterns.
   C. monitor the cough reflex.
   D. instruct the client in the use of throat lozenges.

6. Posterior nosebleeds are usually associated with secondary systemic disorders. The individual most affected by this form of epistaxis is the:
   A. 30-year-old football player.
   B. 62-year-old housewife.
   C. 14-year-old ballet dancer.
   D. 76-year-old retired engineer.

7. Appropriate first aid for the client with an anterior nosebleed includes:
   A. pinching the nose away from the septum.
   B. applying ice packs to the nose.
   C. sitting position, leaning slightly backward.
   D. tilting the head upward.

8. The most common broken bone of the face is the:
   A. mandible.
   B. maxilla.
   C. nose.
   D. temporal bone.

9. Your client has undergone rhinoplasty and will be discharged from the hospital in two days. He is anxious about the swelling and bruising on his face and asks how long the bruises will be noticeable. You reply that this condition should subside in:
   A. 3–5 days.
   B. 6–10 days.
   C. 10–14 days.
   D. several months.

10. The most common cause of airway obstruction in the adult is:
    A. swollen tongue.
    B. drowning.
    C. anaphylactic shock.
    D. food lodged in the throat.

11. The term used to describe a high-pitched, wheezing sound created by an airway obstruction is called:
    A. crowing.
    B. stridor.
    C. sonorous.
    D. crepitus.

12. Upper airway tumors are most commonly found in the:
    A. trachea.
    B. larynx.
    C. nasopharynx.
    D. oropharynx.

13. Laryngeal cancer may be caused by several factors. The risk factor that is considered to be the most modifiable is:
    A. gender.
    B. age.
    C. nutrition.
    D. smoking.

14. Which of the following is considered the treatment of choice for early laryngeal cancer?
    A. Surgery
    B. Chemotherapy
    C. Radiation therapy
    D. Multiple-drug regimen therapy

15. Your client is scheduled for a total laryngectomy. Which of the following diagnoses would be the most appropriate to place on the written care plan after the surgery?
    A. Imbalanced Nutrition: Less than Body Requirements
    B. Impaired Verbal Communication
    C. Grieving
    D. Risk for Aspiration

Chapter 23

Caring for Clients With Lower Respiratory Disorders

EXPLORE **mynursingkit** ™

MyNursingKit is your one stop for online chapter review materials and resources. Prepare for success with additional NCLEX®-style practice questions, interactive assignments and activities, web links, animations and videos, and more!

Register your access code from the front of your book at
www.mynursingkit.com

KEY TERMS

Match each term with its appropriate definition.

C 1. Barrel chest

H 2. Surfactant

F 3. Intercostal

J 4. Parietal pleura

G 5. Left lung

E 6. Alveoli

D 7. Visceral pleura

A 8. Mediastinum

B 9. Right lung

I 10. Tidal volume

A. Composed of the heart and the great vessels

B. Consists of three lobes

C. Increased anterior-posterior chest diameter

D. Covers the external lung surface

E. Location of oxygen and carbon dioxide exchange

F. Space between the ribs

G. Consists of two lobes

H. Substance that prevents the collapse of the alveoli

I. Amount of air moved with normal breathing

J. Lining of the thoracic wall and mediastinum

LEARNING OUTCOMES

1. Define dyspnea, hemoptysis, and cyanosis.

2. Describe aspiration pneumonia.

3. Identify diagnostic testing for pneumonia.

4. Identify nursing diagnoses for pneumonia.

5. Describe tuberculosis.

6. Define negative and positive TB test results.

7. Define asthma.

8. Describe manifestations of COPD.

9. Define barrel chest.

10. Identify manifestations of lung cancer.

APPLY WHAT YOU LEARNED

A 59-year-old woman on your unit has been diagnosed with a pneumothorax and will have a chest tube inserted for treatment. The client has chronic lung disease and has recently quit smoking. She has family members present who are very supportive and eager to learn how to help.

1. Describe nursing care regarding the chest tube.

2. What nursing diagnoses would the nurse apply to this client?

3. What types of evaluation would the nurse provide?

MULTIPLE CHOICE

Circle the answer that best completes the following statements.

1. The most common cause of chronic obstructive pulmonary disease is:
   A. environmental pollutants.
   B. alpha-1 antitrypsin deficiency.
   C. heredity.
   D. smoking.

2. A nursing assistant asks you why the lower respiratory system is so important. She understands that you have to breathe in order to live but wants to know the physiology. Your best response would be:
   A. "The lower respiratory tract warms the air."
   B. "The bronchi allow carbon dioxide and oxygen exchange."
   C. "The alveoli produce a substance that helps the lungs move freely."
   D. "Oxygen and carbon dioxide exchange helps to regulate the acid–base balance."

3. The nurse is teaching the client about her asthmatic condition. The focus of the nursing plan should be:
   A. preventing death.
   B. controlling symptoms.
   C. preventing the asthma attack.
   D. instructing about the pathophysiology of asthma as a disease.

4. The client with asthma is being evaluated for Ineffective Airway Clearance. Which of the following nursing interventions should be the nurse's highest priority?
   A. Monitor oxygen saturation level
   B. Check the chart for the latest ABG report
   C. Assess respiratory effort
   D. Check the amount and color of sputum

5. Your client is complaining of SOB. As you begin your assessment, you note that only the right side of the chest is moving. Your next action should be to:
   A. call the charge nurse.
   B. ask the client why she is only breathing on one side.
   C. apply oxygen at 3 L/nc.
   D. auscultate both lungs.

6. A client was working in a factory that produced a variety of glues. He presents to the emergency room with SOB, fever, and chest pain. Based on your knowledge of pneumonia, you anticipate that this client might have:
   A. aspiration pneumonia.
   B. *Pneumocystis jiroveci* pneumonia.
   C. tuberculosis.
   D. noninfectious pneumonia.

7. Mr. Jackson will be having a thoracentesis on your shift. If all of the following are appropriate interventions for the client before the procedure, which would have the highest priority?
   A. Tell the client that some pressure will be felt.
   B. Bring the supplies to the bedside.
   C. Administer a cough suppressant, if ordered.
   D. Reinforce teaching about the procedure.

8. The nurse is reading the TB skin test for a client. She measures the redness as 6 mm. This measurement is:
   A. a negative response.
   B. a negative response with no infection.
   C. positive for a person with HIV.
   D. invalid because the induration was not read.

9. Johnny, a 29-year-old HIV client, has been taking INH for 2 months. He is now complaining of numbness in his feet. You explain that:
   A. this is an unusual side effect.
   B. he needs to be taking vitamin B_6 along with the INH.
   C. it is a minor problem and will resolve over time.
   D. it is probably caused by his HIV status.

10. A second-day postoperative client complains of sudden chest pain and SOB. The nurse suspects:
    A. pulmonary embolism.
    B. aspiration pneumonia.
    C. atelectasis.
    D. hemorrhage.

11. You are assessing the chest tube for a client with lung cancer. You notice that the water in the water seal is fluctuating with the client's breathing. Your next action should be to:
    A. continue with the assessment.
    B. call the physician after your assessment.
    C. ask the client if he feels okay.
    D. shake the water chamber to stop the bubbling.

12. A 16-year-old male is brought to the emergency room suffering from a severe headache, nausea, and SOB. His skin has a cherry red appearance. You immediately realize that this client may be experiencing:
    A. carbon monoxide poisoning.
    B. status asthmaticus.
    C. walking pneumonia.
    D. cystic fibrosis.

13. During a football game, a player trips and falls. He is brought to the local clinic complaining of severe SOB, tachypnea, and pallor. You note there is asymmetrical lung expansion. You anticipate the insertion of a(n):
    A. IV line.
    B. Foley catheter.
    C. chest tube.
    D. endotracheal tube.

14. The physician has ordered a sputum sample. The nurse knows that the best time to obtain a sputum sample is:
    A. after the first dose of the antibiotic.
    B. right before bedtime.
    C. early in the morning.
    D. late in the afternoon.

15. You are preparing to suction a tracheostomy patient. You remember from your respiratory class that you can apply suction for:
    A. 10 seconds.
    B. 15 seconds.
    C. 25 seconds.
    D. 30 seconds.

Chapter 24

The Gastrointestinal System and Assessment

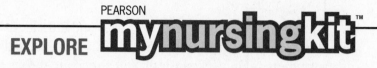

EXPLORE PEARSON mynursingkit™

MyNursingKit is your one stop for online chapter review materials and resources. Prepare for success with additional NCLEX®-style practice questions, interactive assignments and activities, web links, animations and videos, and more!

Register your access code from the front of your book at
www.mynursingkit.com

KEY TERMS

Match each term with its appropriate definition.

E   1. GI tract

A. Metabolizes carbohydrates, proteins, and fats

F   2. Stomach

B. Carries food to the stomach ✓

F   3. Parietal cell

C. Upper opening of the GI tract lined with mucous membranes

J   4. Chief cell

D. Secretes hormones that regulate digestion

H   5. Mucus cell

E. Continuous hollow tube ✓

D   6. Enteroendocrine cell

F. Secretes hydrochloric acid and intrinsic factor

A   7. Liver

G. Contains amylase and lysozymes to break down food

C   8. Mouth

H. Protects the lining of the stomach from gastric juices

G   9. Saliva

I. Connected to the esophagus at the upper end and the small intestine at the lower end ✓

B   10. Esophagus

J. Produces pepsin, which digests protein

LEARNING OUTCOMES

1. Define peristalsis.

2. Explain the components of the gastrointestinal tract.

3. Describe the functions of the liver.

4. Identify the purpose of an upper endoscopy.

5. Discuss the rationale for using imaging studies for gastrointestinal complaints.

6. Describe the diagnostic test called esophageal manometry.

7. Explain the organs located in the right upper quadrant of the abdomen.

8. Identify the purpose of the stool specimen test for ova and parasites.

9. Describe manifestations related to vitamin and mineral deficiencies.

10. Identify symptoms associated with water deficits and excesses.

APPLY WHAT YOU LEARNED

A 45-year-old male presents to your unit with complaints of abdominal pain that has been progressing over the last four days. He states that he has had diarrhea for about a week and does not really have an appetite.

1. What types of questions should the nurse ask to assess the situation further?

2. In what order would the nurse assess the abdomen?

3. What diagnostic testing would the nurse expect the physician to order?

4. Would the nurse offer this client anything to eat?

MULTIPLE CHOICE

Circle the answer that best completes the following statements.

1. A client suffering from multiple dental caries states, "I've been dieting a lot lately." What type of diet is this client on?
   A. High carbohydrates
   B. Low fat
   C. High protein
   D. Fasting

2. Dianne, a patient in the hospital, has not eaten well in several days. She and her boyfriend broke up before she entered the hospital. The nurse realizes that emotions such as stress or anxiety affect the GI tract by:
   A. increasing gastric secretions.
   B. neutralizing stomach acid.
   C. inhibiting gastric motility.
   D. excreting bile.

3. The nurse is caring for a client with liver cancer. Her main concern at this time would be:
   A. prevention of constipation.
   B. prevention of infection.
   C. prevention of gastric reflux.
   D. prevention of discomfort.

4. A gastric analysis includes which of the following?
   A. Allowing the client to smoke
   B. Inserting an NG tube
   C. Observing for falls
   D. Comparing preanalysis weight

5. Bill is 6'0" and weighs 380 pounds. According to the weight chart he should weigh about 185 pounds. Bill is considered to be:
   A. within the normal range.
   B. overweight.
   C. obese.
   D. morbidly obese.

6. Corey was admitted with diarrhea and dehydration. He has at least four foul-smelling, muous-filled loose stools every three hours. You know the doctor will order a:
   A. serum albumin level.
   B. gastric lavage.
   C. endoscopy.
   D. specimen for ova and parasites.

7. You are explaining smoking cessation to a client diagnosed with pancreatic disease. Your best explanation might be:
   A. "The tar in the cigarette coats the lining of the stomach."
   B. "Smoking increases the production of gastric acid secretion."
   C. "Cigarettes inhibit bicarbonate secretion."
   D. "The nicotine increases blood flow to the gastric mucosa."

8. Mr. Lee, an 89-year-old client who rarely eats his meals, is losing weight. The nurse knows to assess:
   A. mucous membranes and gums.
   B. food tolerance.
   C. A and B.
   D. the soft palate.

9. Ms. Ray has soft, spoon-shaped nails. The nurse is aware that this is due to:
   A. protein deficiency.
   B. high-fat diet.
   C. smoking.
   D. iron deficiency.

10. Mrs. Matherly is returning to your unit following a lower GI series. Which of the following nursing interventions is the most important?
    A. Encourage fluids
    B. Monitor for pain
    C. Provide detailed postop instructions
    D. Encourage splinting

11. Which of the following vitamins is water-soluble?
    A. A
    B. D
    C. E
    D. B

12. Energy that is produced by food is measured in:
    A. metabolic rates.
    B. kilocalories.
    C. resting metabolic rates.
    D. body surface area.

13. When assessing the abdomen, which task is first?
    A. Percussion
    B. Palpation
    C. Auscultation
    D. Injection

14. AST and ALT are used to evaluate:
    A. gastric function.
    B. pancreas function.
    C. liver function.
    D. respiratory function.

15. Which diagnostic test is used to detect bleeding in the peritoneal cavity?
    A. Esophageal manometry
    B. Paracentesis
    C. Barium enema
    D. CT scans

Chapter 25

Caring for Clients With Nutritional and Upper Gastrointestinal Disorders

KEY TERMS

Match each term with its appropriate definition.

J   1.   Chyme   A.   Physical and chemical processes of cell activity

C   2.   Hematemesis   B.   Waves of contractions found in GI tract

F   3.   Nutrition   C.   Bloody emesis

E   4.   Nutrient   D.   Pain or difficulty swallowing

G   5.   Malnutrition   E.   Substance needed for growth, maintenance, and repair

H   6.   Melena   F.   Properties of food that build healthy bodies

A   7.   Metabolism   G.   Poor nourishment from improper diet or metabolic defect

B   8.   Peristalsis   H.   Blood in the stool

D   9.   Dysphagia   I.   Area of GI tract that chemically breaks down and absorbs food

I   10. Small intestine   J.   Partially digested food with gastric juices

LEARNING OUTCOMES

1. Define obesity and morbid obesity.

2. Identify some problems associated with obesity.

3. Describe behavior strategies for weight loss.

4. Discuss conditions associated with malnutrition.

5. Define catabolism.

6. Explain the purpose of enteral feedings.

7. Describe anorexia nervosa.

8. Define stomatitis.

9. Identify manifestations regarding oral cancer.

10. Describe gastroesophageal reflux.

APPLY WHAT YOU LEARNED

A client comes to you stating that they are prepared to have a gastric bypass to assist with weight loss and to improve their overall health. The client is categorized as morbidly obese and qualifies for the procedure. The client has documentation from a dietitian regarding past weight loss efforts. The client has also been screened by a psychiatrist to rule out disordered eating and thinking.

1. What educational topics must the nurse discuss with the client before the surgeon obtains consent?

2. What side effects should the nurse explain to the client regarding after-care?

3. What would be the priorities in nursing care regarding this client?

MULTIPLE CHOICE

Circle the answer that best completes the following statements.

1. A client suffering from bulimia is at risk for:
   A. weight gain.
   B. diarrhea.
   C. esophageal damage.
   D. hyperglycemia.

2. Johnny is going to be receiving enteral tube feedings for a period of time. You know that enteral feedings may be administered through:
   A. nasogastric and gastric tubes.
   B. gastric and cecum tubes.
   C. gastric tubes only.
   D. nasogastric, gastrostomy, and jejunostomy tubes.

3. The nurse is caring for a stroke patient receiving 120 mL Ensure/hour. Her main concern at this time would be:
   A. prevention of diarrhea.
   B. prevention of aspiration.
   C. prevention of nasal irritation.
   D. prevention of constipation.

4. A client receiving TPN would be expected to have daily blood specimens drawn for:
   A. calcium.
   B. glucose.
   C. sodium.
   D. potassium.

5. Mary is 5'6" and weighs 160 pounds. According to the weight chart she should weigh about 145 pounds. Mary is considered to be:
   A. within the normal range.
   B. overweight.
   C. obese.
   D. morbidly obese.

6. Maxine was admitted with acute gastritis. During her morning bath, she suddenly begins to throw up blood. Your first action should be to:
   A. administer prescribed antiemetic.
   B. raise the head of the bed.
   C. increase the IV fluid rate.
   D. call the physician.

7. You are explaining to a client who has been diagnosed with peptic ulcer disease the effects that cigarette smoking has on the stomach. Your best explanation might be:
   A. "The tar in the cigarette coats the lining of the stomach."
   B. "Smoking increases the production of gastric acid secretion."
   C. "Cigarettes inhibit bicarbonate secretion."
   D. "The nicotine increases blood flow to the gastric mucosa."

8. Mr. Jessup tells you that he becomes nauseated about 10 minutes after he has eaten. In addition, he states that his stomach cramps and makes loud noises. To alleviate some of these symptoms, the nurse would suggest:
   A. Eat two large meals a day.
   B. Drink lots of water with the food.
   C. Rest in a recumbent position after eating.
   D. Increase the amount of simple sugars in the diet.

9. The nurse is aware that there is an increased risk for stomach cancer in clients who:
   A. eat diets high in fiber.
   B. have been diagnosed with *H. pylori*.
   C. are under a lot of stress.
   D. smoke two packs of cigarettes per day.

10. Mrs. Elliot is returning to your unit following an endoscopy. Which of the following nursing interventions is the most important?
    A. Withhold fluids until the gag reflex returns.
    B. Monitor for pain.
    C. Provide detailed discharge instructions.
    D. Discourage coughing.

11. You are performing a gastric lavage and have suctioned 135 mL of fluid from the stomach. Your initial irrigation was 100 mL of water. On the I&O record you will document:
    A. 135 mL gastric contents.
    B. 235 mL gastric contents and lavage.
    C. 35 mL gastric contents.
    D. 100 mL gastric contents.

12. Mrs. Tubbman has a new gastrostomy tube that is going to be used for the first time. You are unable to aspirate any stomach contents. Bowel sounds are absent. Your next action is to:
    A. use the tube because the x-ray verified placement.
    B. hold the tube feeding until the doctor makes rounds.
    C. call the doctor and inform him of your findings.
    D. ask the charge nurse to begin the feedings.

13. You are teaching a client about the use of metoclopramide. Which of the following is not true concerning this medication?
    A. May cause drowsiness
    B. Used to prevent dizzy spells
    C. Adverse reactions with alcohol have been documented
    D. May have a side effect of muscle tremors

14. The school nurse is seeing an 18-year-old girl for complaints of fatigue. The client states that her vitamins "just don't seem to work." She appears unusually thin. The nurse believes that the client needs further teaching because:
    A. teenagers are not nutritionally educated.
    B. teen girls are at risk for poor nutrition due to societal expectations.
    C. she is on the basketball team and weight loss is expected.
    D. she is not taking the proper amount of vitamins.

15. Measures that are used to evaluate obesity include:
    A. BMI.
    B. fat-fold.
    C. bioelectrical impedance.
    D. all of the above.

Chapter 26

Caring for Clients With Bowel Disorders

KEY TERMS

Match each term with its appropriate definition.

C   1.   Duodenum   A.   Cells located in the intestinal tract that produce mucus

E   2.   Chyme   B.   Outlet of the rectum

H   3.   Ileocecal valve   C.   First part of the large [small] intestine

J   4.   Sigmoid colon   D.   Body waste

D   5.   Feces   E.   Mixture of partly digested food and digestive secretions

I   6.   Defecation reflex   F.   Bearing-down movement

F   7.   Valsalva's maneuver   G.   Worm-shaped pouch extending from the cecum

A   8.   Goblet cells   H.   Connects the small and large intestines

G   9.   Appendix   I.   Stimulation of stretch receptors to allow evacuation

B   10.   Anus   J.   S-shaped portion at the end of the descending colon

LEARNING OUTCOMES

1. Describe the pathophysiology of diarrhea.

2. Identify the foods that may aggravate chronic diarrhea.

3. Discuss preventive measures for constipation in the older adult.

4. Describe the various types of enemas.

5. Define IBS.

6. Discuss nursing care regarding a small bowel series.

7. Define malabsorption.

8. Describe the manifestations of peritonitis.

9. Discuss the diagnostic testing for Crohn's disease.

10. Identify risk factors for colorectal cancer.

APPLY WHAT YOU LEARNED

A client is seen for a follow-up due to a recent hospitalization for IBD. She states that she is feeling better and is slowly advancing her diet from liquids to soft foods that are low in fat. She currently denies diarrhea, constipation, and pain.

Upon assessment, you notice that her abdomen is slightly distended and her blood pressure is 110/78.

1. What nursing diagnoses would apply to this client?

2. Based on the information above, is this normal or abnormal? Why or why not?

3. Explain some teaching the nurse could provide to this client.

MULTIPLE CHOICE

Circle the answer that best completes the following statements.

1. The nurse is changing an ostomy pouch. Which of the following should be completed first?
    A. Note the color of the stoma and surrounding skin.
    B. Use a measuring guide to check stoma size.
    C. Remove the soiled pouch.
    D. Cleanse the skin with soap and water.

2. You are assisting an elderly client in filling out the diet menu. The client has chronic diarrhea. Which of the following items should not be ordered for this client?
    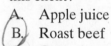
    A. Apple juice
    B. Roast beef
    C. Green beans
    D. Spaghetti

3. The nurse would question the medication order for a client taking a monoamine oxidase inhibitor if which of the following were added to the medication record?
    A. Pepto-Bismol
    B. Lomotil
    C. Sandostatin
    D. Dipentum

4. A young client asks the nurse what causes constipation. The best response is:
    A. lack of exercise.
    B. chronic laxative use.
    C. voluntary suppression of the urge.
    D. all of the above.

5. A client is preparing for a colonoscopy. The physician orders magnesium citrate. Which of the following statements, if made by the client, would indicate an understanding of your teaching instructions?
    A. "I'll take the medication at bedtime so it has time to work."
    B. "If I keep the drink at room temperature it will taste better."
    C. "This medication will give me some cramps."
    D. "It's okay to eat breakfast at 6 A.M., since my exam isn't until 8 A.M."

6. An elderly client has been taking mineral oil as a laxative routinely for several months. The nurse can expect that this client will have a deficiency of:
    A. vitamin A.
    B. vitamin C.
    C. vitamin B.
    D. vitamin F.

7. When preparing a client for a sigmoidoscopy, the teaching plan should include which of the following instructions?
    A. Sterile water may be injected into the bowel for better visualization.
    B. The client will be placed in the prone position.
    C. No food or water can be consumed 8 hours before the test.
    D. The procedure will take about 15 minutes.

8. The primary purpose for assessing the patency of a nasogastric tube is to:
    A. prevent aspiration pneumonia.
    B. remove gastrointestinal secretions.
    C. assess for the return of peristalsis.
    D. replace electrolytes.

9. Which of the following clients is at high risk for developing colon cancer?
    A. 58-year-old male diagnosed with prostate cancer
    B. 24-year-old female with a family history of ovarian cancer
    C. 37-year-old male with inflammatory bowel disease
    D. 16-year-old female with morbid obesity

10. A client tells you that his colostomy bag odor is embarrassing and asks you what he can do to minimize this problem. Your best response would be:
    A. "Be sure to eat lots of cabbage and eggs."
    B. "There's not much that we can do about the smell."
    C. "There are odor tablets that you can put in the bag."
    D. "I don't think the smell is so bad. Don't worry about it."

11. Which observation of a client who has a nursing diagnosis of Risk for Impaired Skin Integrity would indicate that the outcome is successful?
    A. Client has developed a small, 2 cm reddened area on his sacrum.
    B. Client has a small rash on the perineal area.
    C. Client's skin is intact.
    D. Client requires aloe vera cream for lesion on buttocks.

12. When a client has a nursing diagnosis of Risk for Deficient Fluid Volume, which of the following nursing interventions should be included on the care plan?
    A. Maintain accurate intake and output records.
    B. Record the client's weight weekly.
    C. Assess for signs of dehydration, such as moist skin.
    D. Document the vital signs every shift.

13. Which of the following nursing diagnoses would be the most appropriate for a client with colon cancer?
    A. Acute Pain
    B. Grieving
    C. Risk for Sexual Dysfunction
    D. Risk for Impaired Skin Integrity

14. A client is being discharged from the hospital with a new ostomy appliance. Prior to discharge, it is important to request a referral to the:
    A. dietitian.
    B. home health nurse.
    C. ostomy and wound care nurse.
    D. physical therapist.

15. A 24-year-old client is admitted to the surgical floor with excruciating pain in the right groin. He is nauseated and has vomited 300 mL of yellow bile. Visible inspection reveals a mass in the groin. The medical diagnosis for this client might be:
    A. ventral hernia.
    B. strangulated hernia.
    C. umbilical hernia.
    D. incisional hernia.

Chapter 27

Caring for Clients With Gallbladder, Liver, and Pancreatic Disorders

KEY TERMS

Match each term with its appropriate definition.

G	1. Visceral	A.	Circular muscle found in bile duct
C	2. Hepatocytes	B.	Storage place for bile
E	3. Kupffer	C.	Liver cell
A	4. Sphincter of Oddi	D.	A salt that neutralizes acid
I	5. Lipase	E.	Phagocytic cell in the liver
J	6. Exocrine	F.	Yellow-orange fluid produced in liver
F	7. Bile	G.	Pertaining to any large organ in abdomen
B	8. Gallbladder	H.	Small vascular units in the liver
H	9. Lobules	I.	Fat-splitting enzyme
D	10. Bicarbonate	J.	Gland that secretes via a duct

LEARNING OUTCOMES

1. Identify risk factors for gallstones.

2. Define biliary colic.

3. Describe foods to avoid in cholelithiasis.

4. Describe hepatitis.

5. Define jaundice.

6. Identify people who should be vaccinated for hepatitis B.

7. Describe the pathophysiology of cirrhosis.

8. Identify diagnostic testing for cirrhosis.

9. Discuss manifestations of pancreatitis.

10. Describe lab tests for pancreatic disorders.

APPLY WHAT YOU LEARNED

You are planning the discharge for Mr. W, who has been diagnosed with alcohol-induced cirrhosis. His medications are Aldactone, Riopan, lactulose, and a fluid restriction of 1,500 mL/day. He will return home where he lives with his wife of 28 years. He has two children who are grown and live out of state.

1. What nursing interventions will be implemented?

2. What discharge instructions will the nurse review with the wife?

3. Identify nursing diagnoses for this client.

MULTIPLE CHOICE

Circle the answer that best completes the following statements.

1. You are discussing the various forms of hepatitis with the nursing instructor. She asks you which viral hepatitis is transmitted only by blood. Your response should be:
   A. G.
   B. E.
   C. D.
   D. C.

2. Which prescription would the nurse anticipate for a client who has been diagnosed with cirrhosis of the liver?
   A. Lactulose
   B. Acetaminophen
   C. Ibuprophen
   D. Demerol

3. As a result of a client's positive HIDA scan, the nurse expects his immediate treatment to include:
   A. high-protein diet.
   B. low-protein diet.
   C. high-fat diet.
   D. low-fat diet.

4. A client has been diagnosed with acute pancreatitis. Which of the following complications should be anticipated by the nurse?
   A. Hypertension
   B. Flank bruising
   C. Hypoglycemia
   D. Fever

5. Mr. Blue, 48 years old, is diagnosed with cirrhosis of the liver. Which intervention should the nurse plan to include in the client's skin care?
   A. Rub the skin briskly to aid in the drying process.
   B. Turn the client every 20 minutes.
   C. Use hot water when bathing.
   D. Avoid soap for bathing.

6. You are preparing a client for a paracentesis. Which of the following best explains the procedure?
   A. Fluid is removed from the retroperitoneal cavity.
   B. A long needle is inserted into the retroperitoneal cavity.
   C. A needle is inserted into the peritoneal cavity and fluid is withdrawn.
   D. Fluid is removed from the thoracic cavity via a long needle.

7. The nurse is reviewing the lab results for a client with acute pancreatitis. Which of the following would verify that this diagnosis is correct?
   A. Serum amylase 184 U/L
   B. Serum lipase 10 U/L
   C. Serum calcium 12 mg/dL
   D. WBC 5500

8. A client is receiving spironolactone for treatment of cirrhosis. Which of the following statements, if made by the client, would indicate that he understands the medication teaching?
   A. "I'm going to report any diarrhea to my doctor."
   B. "I should take this medication in the morning."
   C. "If I have any ringing in the ears, I'll call you."
   D. "I'll weigh myself every other day."

9. A client returns from surgery with a T-tube. Which of the following interventions would not be appropriate for this client?
   A. Place in Fowler's position.
   B. Keep the T-tube clamped.
   C. Monitor color and consistency of drainage.
   D. Assess skin for bile leakage.

10. When assessing a client in the preicteric phase of acute viral hepatitis, the nurse would expect to identify which of these symptoms?
    A. Pruritus
    B. Clay-colored stools
    C. Flulike symptoms
    D. Increased energy

11. A client with acute hepatitis is experiencing anorexia and nausea. These signs would substantiate a nursing diagnosis of:
    A. Self-Care Deficit.
    B. Activity Intolerance.
    C. Risk for Infection.
    D. Altered Nutrition: Less than Body Requirements.

12. Which of these events, if present in a client's history, is most likely related to the development of hepatitis?
    A. Injection drug user
    B. Recent travel to Florida
    C. Viral infection of the upper airway
    D. History of flu vaccine

13. You are assisting in a liver biopsy. If all of the following are postprocedure nursing interventions, which should be your highest priority?
    A. Position the client on his right side.
    B. Keep NPO for two hours.
    C. Frequently assess site.
    D. Apply direct pressure after the needle is removed.

14. The nurse is teaching a client about the importance of bleeding precautions. Which of the following should not be included in the care plan?
    A. Avoid blowing nose.
    B. Use a medium-hard toothbrush.
    C. Assess for purpura.
    D. Avoid injections.

15. Lactulose is frequently used in the treatment of hepatic encephalopathy. The purpose of this medication is to:
    A. inhibit ammonia absorption in the bowel.
    B. destroy intestinal bacteria.
    C. reduce ascites.
    D. reduce peristalsis.

Chapter 28

The Urinary System and Assessment

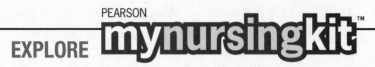

EXPLORE PEARSON mynursingkit™

MyNursingKit is your one stop for online chapter review materials and resources. Prepare for success with additional NCLEX®-style practice questions, interactive assignments and activities, web links, animations and videos, and more!

Register your access code from the front of your book at **www.mynursingkit.com**

KEY TERMS

Match each term with its appropriate definition.

D __ 1. Glomeruli   A. Chief end product of protein metabolism

C __ 2. Nephrons   B. Formed in muscle and excreted in the urine

F __ 3. Ureters   C. Functional units of the kidney

H __ 4. Urinary meatus   D. Small clusters of capillaries

E __ 5. GFR   E. Rate at which blood is filtered in the glomeruli

I __ 6. Urethra   F. Tubes that move urine from the kidneys to the bladder by peristaltic waves

G __ 7. Proximal tubules   G. Small channels that begin the filtration process

J __ 8. Renin   H. Opening of urinary path to the outside of the body

A __ 9. Urea   I. Tube that carries urine outside of the body

B __ 10. Creatinine   J. Plays a role in the regulation of blood pressure

LEARNING OUTCOMES

1. Define nephrons.

2. Describe the function of the ureters.

3. Describe the glomerular filtration process.

4. Identify the normal glomerular filtration rate.

5. Discuss the differences between dysuria, nocturia, and hematuria.

6. Identify laboratory tests commonly used to evaluate renal function.

7. Define uroflowmetry.

8. Describe the 24-hour urine specimen process.

9. Identify teaching points regarding a cystoscopy.

10. Describe components involved in urine studies.

APPLY WHAT YOU LEARNED

A newly admitted male client is being tested because of complaints related to pain upon urination. The client is offering vague descriptions of his symptoms. The physician has ordered blood work and a 24-hour urine test along with some imaging studies.

1. Describe the procedure involved with a 24-hour urine specimen collection.

2. What imaging studies will be done for this client?

3. What is the physician looking for in the blood work related to kidney function?

MULTIPLE CHOICE

Circle the answer that best completes the following statements.

1. Your client has been ordered to have a post-void residual catheterization. Which of the following statements made by the client indicates understanding of the procedure?
   A. "I will call you after I have gone to the bathroom and urinated."
   B. "I will be sure to flush the toilet after I have voided."
   C. "As soon as I void, the nurse will catheterize me."
   D. "The nurse will leave the catheter in place after the procedure."

2. When obtaining a health history from Katie about her urinary status, the nurse asks the following questions except:
   A. "Are you going to the bathroom frequently?"
   B. "Have you noticed blood in your urine?"
   C. "Do you have a discharge from your vagina after intercourse?"
   D. "What is your fluid intake during the day?"

3. In a renal clearance there are two substances found in the blood that are routinely used to evaluate renal function. The effective indicators of renal function are:
   A. blood urea and GFR.
   B. BUN and serum creatinine.
   C. GFR and BUN.
   D. uric acid levels and creatinine.

4. You are asked to obtain a sterile urine sample from an elderly client with dementia. The first action should be to:
   A. cleanse the perineal area.
   B. label the container.
   C. place the client in the dorsal recumbent position.
   D. obtain all the supplies needed.

5. A 24-hour urine test is also known as a:
   A. blood urea nitrogen test.
   B. GFR.
   C. creatinine clearance test.
   D. KUB.

6. The physician has ordered a 24-hour urine test for a client with renal disease. The test is to begin at 6 A.M. At what time should the client empty his bladder and discard the urine?
   A. 5 A.M.
   B. 5:30 A.M.
   C. 6 A.M.
   D. The client does not discard any urine.

7. Nursing care for the client to evaluate urinary retention and incontinence includes all of the following except:
   A. administering pain medications.
   B. using an uroflowmeter.
   C. obtaining a specimen.
   D. measuring urine output.

8. A urinalysis has just been received on the unit for Mr. Kattes. The nurse is aware that a normal urinalysis should not have:
   A. ketones—negative.
   B. protein—3+.
   C. WBC—0–5/HPF.
   D. glucose—negative.

9. Ultrasound examination of the bladder or kidneys is a noninvasive examination that requires:
   A. the client to ingest dye to see the organs.
   B. an empty stomach.
   C. no preparation of the client.
   D. a full bladder.

10. When teaching a client about a renal scan, the nurse informs her that she must increase fluid intake:
    A. before and after the scan.
    B. four hours before the scan.
    C. after the scan only.
    D. before the scan only.

11. The functional unit of the kidney is known as the:
    A. ureter.
    B. nephron.
    C. urethra.
    D. glomerulus.

12. The nurse understands the normal GFR in adults is:
    A. 50–75 mL/min.
    B. 100–200 mL/min.
    C. 120–125 mL/min.
    D. 10–15 mL/min.

13. Foul-smelling urine with a cloudy appearance is known as:
    A. nocturia.
    B. hematuria.
    C. dysuria.
    D. pyuria.

14. Direct visualization of the urethra and bladder is:
    A. cystoscopy.
    B. renal scan.
    C. ultrasound.
    D. computed tomography.

15. Urine is concentrated in which structure of the kidney?
    A. Loop of Henle
    B. Ureter
    C. Urethra
    D. Bladder

Chapter 29

Caring for Clients With Renal and Urinary Tract Disorders

KEY TERMS

Match each term with its appropriate definition.

C   1.   Incontinence   A.   Pelvic floor muscle exercises

E   2.   Retention   B.   An inflammatory disorder affecting the renal pelvis

A   3.   Kegel   C.   Involuntary urination

G   4.   Credé method   D.   Increased blood levels of nitrogenous wastes, including urea and creatinine

I   5.   Cystitis   E.   Disruption to normal urine flow

B   6.   Pyelonephritis   F.   The most common cause of obstructed urine flow

J   7.   Glomerulonephritis   G.   Applying pressure over the symphysis pubis with the fingers of one or both hands to promote complete bladder emptying

D   8.   Azotemia   H.   Damage to glomerular membranes and severe protein loss in the urine

H   9.   Nephrotic syndrome   I.   The most common UTI

F   10.   Urolithiasis   J.   May be an acute or a chronic disorder

LEARNING OUTCOMES

1. Define urinary incontinence.

2. Identify the types of incontinence.

3. Identify manifestations of urinary tract infections in older adults.

4. Define azotemia.

5. Describe manifestations of urinary stones.

6. Identify foods that are high in purines.

7. Describe nursing diagnoses related to bladder cancer.

8. Define dialysis.

9. Describe renal failure.

10. Discuss implementations of nursing care for excess fluid volume.

APPLY WHAT YOU LEARNED

You are caring for a 72-year-old female with renal failure. The physician has ordered dialysis. The client will be having an arteriovenous fistula placed in the morning. She has a strong support system with many family members including her spouse. Her psychosocial assessment reveals a poor understanding of her condition.

1. How would the nurse describe renal failure to this client and her family to ensure understanding?

2. Describe the process of dialysis.

3. What are some nursing diagnoses that apply to this client?

MULTIPLE CHOICE

Circle the answer that best completes the following statements.

1. Which of the following is the most important point to remember when performing a urinary catheterization?
   A. Assess the amount and color of the initial drainage.
   B. Provide perineal care before performing the procedure.
   C. Use sterile technique when inserting the catheter.
   D. Do not drain more than 800 mL of urine from the bladder.

2. A middle-aged female client is having a minor problem with stress incontinence. Which of the following nursing interventions would not be included in the nursing care plan?
   A. Monitor intake and output.
   B. Teach Kegel exercises.
   C. Try to hold urine as long as possible before going to the bathroom.
   D. Limit beverages after the evening meal.

3. The nurse is teaching a young female how to decrease the risk for a UTI. If all of the following are true, which statement should have the highest priority?
   A. Do not use bubble bath.
   B. Wipe from front to back.
   C. Wipe from back to front.
   D. Empty the bladder at least every two hours.

4. A client asks the nurse about complementary therapies for preventing a UTI. Which of the following fruits would be recommended for this client?
   A. Blueberries
   B. Grape juice
   C. Oranges
   D. Pineapple

5. A 28-year-old client has been admitted to the orthopedic floor after sustaining multiple rib fractures in a motorcycle accident. The physician should be notified if the client develops:
   A. bruising on the chest wall.
   B. a fever of 100 degrees.
   C. oliguria.
   D. an increased appetite.

6. A client receiving Gantrisin for a UTI has developed a rash several hours after taking the first dose. The nurse's best response to this development is:
   A. "The rash is normal. It will go away in a few days."
   B. "You didn't tell me that you were allergic to a sulfa drug!"
   C. "Don't take any more of the medication. I will notify the doctor."
   D. "I should have looked at your chart before I gave you the mediation."

7. Which of the following should be included in the teaching plan for a client with an order for Pyridium?
   A. Take the medication for at least three days.
   B. Take the drug on an empty stomach.
   C. The medication will clear up the infection in one week.
   D. Wear a peripad to protect your underwear.

8. A client has been ordered a low-purine diet. The dietary department calls you to confirm the choices made on the menu. You realize that your client needs further teaching because he ordered:
   A. crab.
   B. tuna.
   C. fried trout.
   D. liver.

9. Which symptom is the client with bladder cancer most likely to exhibit?
   A. Painless hematuria
   B. Urinary frequency
   C. Dysuria
   D. Back pain

10. A client has been admitted for major trauma to the pelvis. The physician tells you that she is hypovolemic and orders an IV NS at 150 mL/hour. Based on this information, you should monitor closely for signs of:
    A. acute renal failure.
    B. spontaneous pneumothorax.
    C. chronic renal failure.
    D. urolithiasis.

11. Which type of incontinence is brought on by sneezing, laughing, or lifting?
    A. Stress
    B. Urge
    C. Overflow
    D. Reflex

12. The nurse understands what about incontinence?
    A. It is a normal part of the aging process.
    B. All people over 65 have some form of it.
    C. It is not a normal part of the aging process.
    D. It only affects people over 80.

13. Condition occurring when trauma interferes with the normal mechanisms of bladder emptying is known as:
    A. neurogenic bladder.
    B. spastic bladder.
    C. benign prostatic hypertrophy.
    D. cystitis.

14. Which of the following is not a manifestation of cystitis?
    A. Dysuria
    B. Hematuria
    C. Incontinence
    D. Frequency

15. A removal of the entire urinary bladder and surrounding tissues is known as:
    A. ileal conduit.
    B. radical cystectomy.
    C. partial cystectomy.
    D. cutaneous ureterostomy.

Chapter 30

The Reproductive System and Assessment

EXPLORE **mynursingkit**
PEARSON

MyNursingKit is your one stop for online chapter review materials and resources. Prepare for success with additional NCLEX®-style practice questions, interactive assignments and activities, web links, animations and videos, and more!

Register your access code from the front of your book at
www.mynursingkit.com

KEY TERMS

Match each term with its appropriate definition.

A   1. Testes
D   2. Scrotum
E   3. Spermatogenesis

G   4. Epididymis

F   5. Testosterone
B   6. Ovaries
I   7. Estrogen

J   8. Progesterone
H   9. Fallopian tubes

C   10. Uterus

A. Produce sperm and testosterone
B. Produce the female hormones
C. Thick-walled, pear-shaped organ in the female, located between the bladder and the rectum
D. Pouch that regulates the temperature of the testes
E. Sperm production
F. Male sex hormone
G. Cordlike structure that provides storage of sperm
H. Excretory duct of the testes
I. Steroid hormone essential to the development and maintenance of secondary sex characteristics
J. Hormone that affects breast glandular tissue and the endometrium

LEARNING OUTCOMES

1. Identify the structures of the male reproductive system.

2. Identify the internal structures of the female reproductive system.

3. Define estrogens.

4. Describe the purpose of mammography.

5. Describe the pelvic ultrasound.

6. Discuss transrectal ultrasonography.

7. Describe the prostate gland.

8. Describe the phases of the ovarian cycle.

9. Define spermatogenesis.

10. Describe seminal fluid.

APPLY WHAT YOU LEARNED

An adolescent presented in the clinic with the onset of her first period. The student nurse is currently studying reproduction and knows that this is a sensitive subject for teen girls to discuss. The client's mother is not with her and she does not know that this is the beginning of a cycle into womanhood.

1. Explain the menstrual cycle.

2. How would the nurse comfort this client and ensure her dignity?

MULTIPLE CHOICE

Circle the answer that best completes the following statements.

1. While palpating the inguinal and groin areas of her male client the nurse knows she is checking for a possible:
   A. STI.
   B. BPH.
   C. hernia.
   D. testicular injury.

2. The nurse knows that when palpating the breast for discharge, the nipples must be
   A. pinched.
   B. rolled.
   C. pulled.
   D. compressed.

3. What is the correct position of a female while her vagina is being assessed?
   A. Supine
   B. Lithotomy
   C. Semi-Fowler's
   D. Knees to chest

4. Tumors that are too small to be detected by clinical breast exam or self-breast exam can be identified by:
   A. mammography.
   B. x-ray.
   C. CT scan.
   D. MRI.

5. When teaching a client about laparoscopy the nurse must remember to tell the client that the night before the exam she must:
   A. eat.
   B. keep her bladder full.
   C. douche.
   D. discuss the treatment methods with her spouse.

6. Instruct the client having mammography that 5 to 7 days before the exam she must avoid caffeine and:
   A. carbonated drinks.
   B. blueberries.
   C. purines.
   D. methylzanthines.

7. Colposcopy can identify early premalignant changes in cervical tissue, and is performed when abnormal results are found on:
   A. CT.
   B. endoscopy.
   C. Pap smear.
   D. MRI.

8. In men, the urethra and penis both serve as organs for urine elimination and ejaculation of:
   A. sperm.
   B. bacteria.
   C. oocytes.
   D. enzymes.

9. Bill has been complaining of a loss in libido. His serum testosterone level is 500 ng/dL. Normal serum levels are:
   A. 650–2000 ng/dL.
   B. 280–1100 ng/dL.
   C. 150–500 ng/dL.
   D. 1–50 ng/dL.

10. What could be another possible problem with Bill's loss of libido?
    A. Drinking
    B. Medications
    C. Mental concerns
    D. All of the above

11. The term used to describe male sex hormones is:
    A. scrotum.
    B. testes.
    C. estrogens.
    D. androgens.

12. The outer layer of the uterine wall is:
    A. perimetrium.
    B. myometrium.
    C. endometrium.
    D. endocervical.

13. The nurse knows that the vaginal mucus is bacteriostatic and:
    A. alkaline.
    B. acidic.
    C. phosphoric.
    D. calciumated.

14. The lab test done to evaluate function of the testes and ovaries is:
    A. serum estradiol.
    B. progesterone.
    C. serum testosterone.
    D. follicle-stimulating hormone.

15. CA125 is a marker used to detect which cancer?
    A. Ovarian
    B. Breast
    C. Testicular
    D. Uterine

Chapter 31

Caring for Male Clients With Reproductive System Disorders

KEY TERMS

Match each term with its appropriate definition.

D   1. BPH

G   2. Adenocarcinoma

_____ 3. Orchiectomy

_____ 4. Brachytherapy

_____ 5. Prostatitis

_____ 6. Testicular torsion

_____ 7. Cremasteric reflex

_____ 8. Cryptorchidism

_____ 9. Epididymitis

_____ 10. Orchitis

A. Can occur as a complication of mumps

B. Failure of one or both testes to descend through the inguinal ring into the scrotum

C. Implants of radioactive seeds

D. Enlargement of the prostate gland

E. Removal of the testes

F. Usually caused by an infection spread from the bladder, urethra, prostate gland, or seminal vesicles

G. Tumor arising from glandular epithelial cells

H. Retraction of the testicles when the skin on the inside of the thigh is stroked

I. Often associated with lower urinary tract infections

J. Twisting of the testes and spermatic cord

LEARNING OUTCOMES

1. Define BPH.

2. Identify manifestations of prostate cancer.

3. Describe diagnostic testing regarding the prostate.

4. Define orchiectomy.

5. Describe the three approaches to a prostatectomy.

6. Identify nursing diagnoses related to prostate dysfunction.

7. Define testicular torsion.

8. Describe cryptorchidism.

9. Discuss testicular cancer.

10. Define erectile dysfunction.

APPLY WHAT YOU LEARNED

A 61-year-old male client presents to your clinic with complaints of urgency regarding urination. During the physical exam, the physician palpates a hard nodule on the prostate gland. Upon further assessment, he tells the physician that he has been getting up three or four times a night to use the bathroom and not much urine comes out when he tries.

1. What diagnostic testing would the nurse expect the physician to order to follow up on the nodule?

2. Would this client be a candidate for a surgical procedure? If so, which one?

3. Describe some teaching that the nurse would do with the client and his wife.

MULTIPLE CHOICE

Circle the answer that best completes the following statements.

1. The nurse has instructed a male client in testicular self-examination. Further teaching is required when the client says:
   A. "The day I do the exam should be the same day each month."
   B. "I should perform the exam in the shower."
   C. "My testicles should feel soft and walnut-size."
   D. "I will check myself before I have sexual intercourse."

2. You are bathing a male client and notice that he is not circumcised. You pull back the foreskin. After you have cleansed the penis, which of the following must be done?
   A. Have the client empty his bladder.
   B. Replace the foreskin.
   C. Clean the anal area.
   D. Document the bath on the nursing notes.

3. Which of the following clients has an increased risk of developing priapism?
   A. 22-year-old male with spinal cord trauma
   B. 35-year-old male with testicular injury
   C. 62-year-old male with BPH
   D. 84-year-old male with impotence

4. The nursing assistant reports that Mr. Peterson has a sore on his penis. He denies any pain. Your best response should be:
   A. "Okay, just be sure and wash him real well."
   B. "I'll be there in a few minutes to take a look at the sore."
   C. "It's probably nothing. Just document it on the nurse's notes."
   D. "It's probably cancer. I'll let the doctor know right away."

5. A client has been diagnosed with erectile dysfunction. If all of the following are appropriate nursing interventions, which should have the highest priority?
   A. Actively listen to your client's concerns.
   B. Teach the client about the condition.
   C. Explain to the client the importance of pelvic floor exercises.
   D. Discuss the treatment methods.

6. When preparing a client for a transrectal ultrasound-guided biopsy of the prostate, the teaching plan should include which of these instructions?
   A. Client will be fully unconscious during the procedure.
   B. An informed consent is not necessary.
   C. Hematuria and bloody streaks are expected several days after the procedure.
   D. Advise the client to continue on his daily dose of aspirin.

7. Which of these statements, if made by the client diagnosed with prostate cancer, would support a nursing diagnosis of Deficient Knowledge?
   A. "There isn't much hope for me, is there?"
   B. "My doctor said I might have some impotence problems after my surgery."
   C. "The hormone therapy won't cure my cancer."
   D. "If I don't get treated, my cancer might go to my lungs."

8. A client is being treated for prostatitis. The nurse should include which of the following diagnoses in the care plan?
   A. Ineffective Protection related to depressed immune system
   B. Fear related to possible death
   C. Activity Intolerance related to fatigue
   D. Disturbed Body Image related to physical changes

9. The nurse is explaining various approaches to a prostatectomy. She would be correct in stating that a suprapubic prostatectomy is done through:
   A. an incision between the scrotum and anus.
   B. an abdominal incision into the bladder.
   C. an abdominal incision with the bladder remaining intact.
   D. an insertion of a Foley catheter.

10. A client is receiving Viagra. The nurse should plan to observe for side effects, which include:
    A. phimosis.
    B. hypertension.
    C. hypokalemia.
    D. hypotension.

11. Which of these measures should be included in the care plan for a client who is recovering from a TURP?
    A. Use clean technique when handling the drainage system.
    B. Frequently assess catheter patency.
    C. Obtain intake and output every 24 hours.
    D. Maintain the CBI to keep the output cherry red.

12. A client presents with complaints that he has no sexual desire. You anticipate that the physician may order a:
    A. psychologic consult.
    B. testosterone level.
    C. routine urinalysis.
    D. PSA.

13. A client asks you what complementary therapies are available for BPH. Your best response should be:
    A. "I can't talk about other treatments, that's the doctor's job."
    B. "Yoga can help you to relax."
    C. "Saw palmetto grass has been known to reduce the symptoms."
    D. "Flomax helps to relax the smooth muscle."

14. Which nursing intervention would be the most appropriate to meet the expected outcome of "client will wake up less frequently during the night" for a client who has BPH?
    A. Advise client to restrict alcohol intake.
    B. Provide information about his condition.
    C. Determine his level of anxiety.
    D. Provide pain measures during the day.

15. The client who is at the highest risk for orchitis is the:
    A. 10-year-old male with measles.
    B. 38-year-old male with HIV.
    C. 42-year-old male with prostate cancer.
    D. 48-year-old male with mumps.

Chapter 32

Caring for Female Clients With Reproductive System Disorders

KEY TERMS

Match each term with its appropriate definition.

_____ 1. Climacteric   A. Pain associated with menstruation

_____ 2. Dyspareunia   B. Period during which menstruation permanently ceases

___A___ 3. PMS   C. Benign uterine or cervical tumors

_____ 4. Dysmenorrhea   D. Pain during sexual intercourse

_____ 5. DUB   E. Vaginal bleeding that is abnormal in amount, duration, or time of occurrence

___H___ 6. Hysterectomy   F. A symptom complex of irritability, depression, edema, and breast tenderness preceding menses

_____ 7. Endometriosis   G. Excessive hair growth

_____ 8. Polycystic ovary syndrome (PCOS)   H. Removal of the uterus

___G___ 9. Hirsutism   I. An endocrine disorder in which LH, estrogen, and androgen hormone levels are higher than normal, and FSH levels are low

___C___ 10. Fibroids   J. Endometrial tissue found outside the uterus

LEARNING OUTCOMES

1. Define menopause.

2. Describe hormone replacement therapy.

3. Discuss premenstrual syndrome.

4. Define hysterectomy.

5. Describe endometriosis.

6. Identify diagnostic testing related to ovarian cysts.

7. Define vaginitis.

8. Describe pelvic inflammatory disease.

9. Discuss cervical cancer.

10. Define uterine prolapse.

APPLY WHAT YOU LEARNED

A 35-year-old female comes into the ER with complaints of nipple discharge, breast pain, and a persistent skin rash near the nipple. She states it started about one week ago and she was going to wait to see if it cleared up on its own. She is not due for her yearly gynecological exam and has not had a mammogram at this point in her life. She states that three of her aunts on her mother's side have had breast cancer.

1. What risk factors does this client have that would make the nurse suspect breast cancer?

2. What diagnostic testing is done to confirm breast cancer?

3. Identify nursing diagnoses related to this client.

4. Describe the grieving process regarding this situation.

MULTIPLE CHOICE

Circle the answer that best completes the following statements.

1. The nurse is teaching a group of middle school girls the signs of breast cancer. Which of the following would she not include in the lecture?
   A. Nipple discharge
   B. Unusual lump in the axilla
   C. Small, hard, painless lump in the breast
   D. Brown area around the nipple

2. A client who is scheduled for a core-needle biopsy may need further instruction if she says:
   A. "The doctor will numb my breast."
   B. "I will lie on my back during the procedure."
   C. "Some of my breast tissue will be removed using a needle."
   D. "I can take a mild painkiller when I go home."

3. You are explaining to your client why she has a swollen abdomen and pain in her upper arm following a laparoscopy. The best explanation would be:
   A. "Carbon monoxide is blown into the abdominal cavity."
   B. "The pain is coming from the surgical incision site."
   C. "The surgeon had to insert a larger instrument to see inside the abdomen."
   D. "It is caused by carbon dioxide. It allows better visualization of internal organs."

4. A 52-year-old client is upset about the onset of menopause. She asks the nurse how she can cope with the symptoms. The best response should be:
   A. "Avoid drinking alcohol or caffeine."
   B. "Everyone has to go through these changes."
   C. "Splash your face with warm water to relax your muscles."
   D. "Keep the room warm, especially at night."

5. The nurse is assisting the physician in obtaining a cervical smear. She knows that the client should be placed in which position?
   A. Sims'
   B. Lithotomy
   C. Supine
   D. Side-lying

6. A client presents to the emergency room with a temperature of 103°F and vomiting. Your assessment reveals hypotension and peeling skin on her palms and feet. There is a foul-smelling discharge from her vagina. The client states that she is on her menses and has a tampon in place. Your next action would be to:
   A. place the client in the lithotomy position.
   B. ask the client to remove the tampon.
   C. ask the client if she is pregnant.
   D. remove the tampon.

7. The nurse recognizes that which factor in the client's history is the most important etiological factor in developing cervical cancer?
   A. Intercourse using a latex condom
   B. Monogamous relationship
   C. Infection with HPV
   D. Poor hygiene

8. Tamoxifen is most often used for the client with breast cancer because it:
   A. inhibits growth of the tumor by blocking estrogen receptor sites.
   B. replaces lost estrogen needed for cancer protection.
   C. reduces the risk of endometrial cancer.
   D. decreases the spread of breast cancer.

9. A client tells the nurse that she has a fishy-smelling, "milk-like" discharge from her vagina. The nurse suspects that this client has:
   A. atrophic vaginitis.
   B. candidiasis.
   C. trichomoniasis.
   D. simple vaginitis.

10. Which of the following clients is most likely to develop breast cancer in her lifetime?
    A. A client with a familial history of colon cancer
    B. A client who started her menstrual period at 14 years of age
    C. A client who had multiple chest x-rays before she was 30 years old
    D. A client who had her first child at the age of 22

11. Upon admission to the medical floor, the nurse should give highest priority to meeting which need of a client diagnosed with PID?
    A. Information related to the prevention of PID
    B. Pain control
    C. Insertion of a Foley catheter
    D. Ordering the daily meals

12. A postmastectomy client refuses to raise her arm above her head because of the presence of a JP drain. The nurse should tell the client:
    A. "You have to exercise your arm to keep it from getting stiff."
    B. "I know it is painful, but the arm needs limbering up."
    C. "You are right. You need to wait until the drains are out to raise your arm."
    D. "Let me get you some pain medication first."

13. In preparing a care plan for a client diagnosed with dysfunctional uterine bleeding, it is most important for the nurse to include a goal that addresses the need for:
    A. sexual function concerns.
    B. increased compliance with the medication regime.
    C. information on how to promote conception.
    D. wound care management.

14. A client has been told that abnormal cells were seen in her initial Pap test. The next action taken by the nurse should be to:
    A. prepare the client for a hysterectomy.
    B. ask the client if she has any questions about the repeat Pap test.
    C. begin an IV of NS in preparation for cauterization of the abnormal cells.
    D. ask the client to sign another consent form.

15. The physician suspects that a client has ovarian cancer. Which of the following lab tests might be ordered to confirm the diagnosis?
    A. PSA
    B. CA 125
    C. WBC
    D. HGB

Chapter 33

Caring for Clients With Sexually Transmitted Infections

KEY TERMS

Match each term with its appropriate definition.

_____	1. Abstinence	A.	Painless ulcer
_____	2. HPV	B.	Slang word for gonorrhea
_____	3. Genital herpes	C.	Venereal Disease Research Laboratory
_____	4. Syphilis	D.	Inflammation of the pelvis
_____	5. Prodromal symptoms	E.	Human papilloma virus
_____	6. Zithromax	F.	Spirochete *Treponema pallidum*
_____	7. Clap	G.	Voluntarily refraining from sexual intercourse
_____	8. Chancre	H.	Herpes simplex 2 virus
_____	9. VDRL	I.	Drug used to treat chlamydia
_____	10. PID	J.	Warning signals of an impending outbreak

LEARNING OUTCOMES

1. Define a sexually transmitted infection.

2. Identify risk factors for STIs.

3. Describe chlamydia.

4. Describe the presentation of gonorrhea.

5. Identify nursing diagnoses related to STIs.

6. Discuss the prevention of STIs.

7. Define genital herpes.

8. Describe syphilis.

9. Describe manifestations regarding trichomoniasis.

10. Identify the STIs that are reportable to state and federal agencies.

APPLY WHAT YOU LEARNED

The student nurse is presenting sexual education information to the local high school with the rest of his nursing class. In preparation, the class has numerous handouts, posters, quizzes, and self-assessment tests for the teens. The student nurse feels well-prepared and nervous at the same time due to the sensitive nature of the topic.

1. What interventions could the student nurse use to feel at ease and put the teens at ease?

2. Reporting STIs to state and federal agencies is an important task and is required by all states. The student nurse knows that which STIs must be reported?

3. Which risk factors will the student nurse elaborate on during the discussion with the teens?

MULTIPLE CHOICE

Circle the answer that best completes the following statements.

1. Miss Doyle is examined by the nurse practitioner. The diagnosis is chlamydia. Which of the following interventions would best meet the need for preventing transmission of the organism?
   A. Encourage her partner to get medical attention.
   B. Recommend abstinence while the lesions are healing.
   C. Provide social and emotional support.
   D. Explain the life cycle of chlamydia.

2. A nurse is teaching a sex education class to a group of high school students. To gain a better understanding of their level of knowledge, the nurse asks the students to say the name of the most common STI. The correct response should be:
   A. syphilis.
   B. chlamydia.
   C. gonorrhea.
   D. genital herpes.

3. A client admits that he forgets to take the medication prescribed for his gonorrhea. The most effective method to overcome this noncompliance would be to:
   A. call him on the telephone as a reminder.
   B. make an appointment with his case worker.
   C. provide extensive education about his infection.
   D. administer a single dose of medication as ordered.

4. A young man is seen in the emergency room for a profuse and purulent urethral discharge. It is important that the nurse gather information related to:
   A. previous infections.
   B. all sexual contacts.
   C. a history of bladder infections.
   D. recent sexual contacts.

5. After assessing an 18-year-old client, the nurse makes the diagnosis of Ineffective Health Maintenance. The nurse understands that further teaching is necessary because the client:
   A. has a stable monogamous relationship with her boyfriend.
   B. has never been tested for chlamydia.
   C. has had annual Pap smears.
   D. has multiple sex partners.

6. Mr. Black was diagnosed with gonorrhea and has been treated with a single dose of Rocephin IM. He is given a prescription for doxycycline to take at home. The nurse explains that this combination of antibiotics is prescribed to:
   A. treat any coexisting chlamydial infection.
   B. eliminate resistant strains of gonorrhea.
   C. prevent the development of resistant organisms.
   D. prevent reinfection.

7. Sally Hart has primary syphilis. While caring for her the nurse should:
   A. wear gloves when taking her vital signs.
   B. place the client in isolation.
   C. assess the feet for the presence of blisters.
   D. discuss safer sex practices.

8. The nurse suspects that the client does not understand the disease process of genital herpes when he says:
   A. "As long as I use the medication, I won't infect anyone."
   B. "I have to abstain from having sex when the lesions are present."
   C. "Burow's solution can be used to cleanse the sores."
   D. "I need to purchase some boxer shorts and wear them during the outbreak."

9. A young client tells you that her girlfriend said that "a person would get cancer if they had the papilloma virus." Your best response should be:
   A. "Your girlfriend isn't your doctor."
   B. "There is a greater risk of cervical cancer for those infected with HPV."
   C. "I've never heard of that."
   D. "That idea is just a myth. Just ignore her."

10. A client is being treated for chlamydia. The nurse knows that the teaching has been effective when the client states:
    A. "One injection of penicillin will cure me."
    B. "Use of a spermicidal foam will protect me from further infections."
    C. "Even if I don't get treated, the chlamydia will eventually go away."
    D. "I need to tell my boyfriend so he can get treated."

11. A 24-year-old client tells you that her boyfriend left her because she has genital warts. She says that he "thought they were disgusting." Based on this information the nurse makes a diagnosis of:
    A. Ineffective Individual Coping.
    B. Anxiety.
    C. Risk for Infection.
    D. Disturbed Body Image.

12. You are collecting data from the chart of a client, age 17, in order to assist in the development of the nursing care plan. You note that this client has been pregnant three times. If all of the following are risk factors for contracting an STI, which should be discussed first?
    A. Use of oral contraceptives
    B. Adolescent sexual activity
    C. Multiple sex partners
    D. Unprotected sexual activity

13. The nurse is discussing discharge instructions with a client who has the "clap." The most important point that should be emphasized is:
    A. take all of the prescribed medication.
    B. use a condom for sexual intercourse.
    C. encourage sexual partners to be treated.
    D. return for follow-up appointment.

14. The risk for contracting any STI is directly related to:
    A. the number of sexual partners.
    B. lifestyle.
    C. age.
    D. gender.

15. Which of the following must be reported to the public health department?
    A. Genital herpes
    B. Syphilis
    C. Chlamydia
    D. Trichomoniasis

Chapter 34

The Endocrine System and Assessment

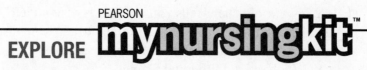

EXPLORE **mynursingkit**™

MyNursingKit is your one stop for online chapter review materials and resources. Prepare for success with additional NCLEX®-style practice questions, interactive assignments and activities, web links, animations and videos, and more!

Register your access code from the front of your book at **www.mynursingkit.com**

KEY TERMS

Match each term with its appropriate definition.

D   1.   Pancreas   A.   Necessary for proper functioning of the thyroid

E   2.   Hypothalamus   B.   Master gland

B   3.   Pituitary   C.   Increases calcium blood levels

G   4.   Adrenal cortex   D.   Secretes digestive enzymes and releases insulin and glucagon into the bloodstream

A   5.   Iodine   E.   Regulates temperature, fluid volume, and growth

F   6.   Islets of Langerhans   F.   Produces insulin

H   7.   Epinephrine   G.   Produces corticosteroids

C   8.   Parathyroid   H.   A counterregulatory hormone

J   9.   Thyroid   I.   Produces hormones known as catecholamines

I   10.   Adrenal medulla   J.   Reduces excess calcium in the blood

LEARNING OUTCOMES

1. Describe the purpose of the endocrine system.

2. Identify the lab tests ordered to diagnose an endocrine disorder.

3. Describe how an MRI is used as a diagnostic tool.

4. Discuss the function of the thyroid gland.

5. Describe the functions of the hypothalamus.

6. Explain the purpose of the pancreas.

7. Identify the purpose of insulin.

8. Describe exophthalmos.

9. Discuss the two hour glucose tolerance test.

10. Explain the purpose of the adrenal cortex.

APPLY WHAT YOU LEARNED

A nursing student is learning about the importance of the endocrine system. Hormones and insulin regulate many parts of the body. While at a clinical rotation, the student is assigned to a client who suffers from Graves' disease.

1. What is Graves' disease?

   Hyperthyroidism

2. How does Graves' disease manifest in the body?

   Bulging Eyes
   Tacycardia
   Intolerence to heat

3. What can the nurse expect for the treatment of this illness?

MULTIPLE CHOICE

Circle the answer that best completes the following statements.

1. A client, diagnosed with diabetes, tells you that he is having increased blood sugars two hours after meals. Based on this statement, the nurse prepares a care plan for a nursing diagnosis of:
   A. Disturbed Body Image related to physical changes.
   B. Activity Intolerance related to increased blood sugars.
   C. Pain related to increased abdominal girth after meals.
   D. Deficient Knowledge related to diagnosis of diabetes.

2. An elderly client is taking a diuretic for mild congestive heart failure. He has recently been admitted to the hospital for SIADH. Which of the following nursing interventions must be included in the plan of care?
   A. Provide oral mouth care at frequent intervals.
   B. Push fluids as tolerated.
   C. Initiate seizure precautions.
   D. Assess respiratory status every 4 hours.

3. Mrs. Leopold presents with a temperature of 99°F, malaise, and says, "I feel tired all the time." Subsequent labs reveal a T_4 of 0.5 mcg/dL. You suspect that Mrs. Leopold will be diagnosed with:
   A. Cushing's syndrome.
   B. severe bronchitis.
   C. hypothyroidism.
   D. sepsis.

4. In the medication instructions for a client taking a corticosteroid, you must include which of the following?
   A. Take the medication on an empty stomach.
   B. Do not stop taking the medication without consulting the physician.
   C. Eat foods that are low in potassium.
   D. Maintain a healthy diet.

5. A common GI complaint for a client diagnosed with hypothyroidism is:
   A. frequent stomach pains.
   B. constipation.
   C. bloody stools.
   D. increased peristalsis.

6. A client complains of an "extreme case of the jitters" and a sensation of thumps in her chest. Her lab values indicate an increased level of T_3 and T_4. Based on this information, the most likely diagnosis will be:
   A. thyrotoxicosis.
   B. cretinism.
   C. hyperparathyroidism.
   D. Cushing's syndrome.

7. A client, diagnosed with diabetes insipidus, is experiencing tachycardia, poor skin turgor, and a dry mouth. The nurse anticipates the development of a care plan for:
   A. nocturia.
   B. polyuria.
   C. dehydration.
   D. hypernatremia.

8. Mrs. Randall comes to the clinic complaining of a wound on her arm that will not heal. During her assessment, she also admits to some difficulty in concentrating, recent weight gain, and fatigue. Your next question is regarding her urine output, because you suspect:
   A. hyperthyroidism.
   B. hypothyroidism.
   C. Cushing's syndrome.
   D. Addison's disease.

9. A client who has recently developed exophthalmos tells you that she has stopped dating. She tells you that she thought her eyes would return to "normal" after her diagnosis of Graves' disease. A primary nursing diagnosis would be:
   A. Ineffective Health Maintenance
   B. Disturbed Personal Identity
   C. Deficient Knowledge
   D. Risk for Situational Low Self-Esteem

10. A client diagnosed with hypoparathyroidism may experience continuous muscle spasms known as:
    A. tetany.
    B. Trousseau.
    C. Chvostek.
    D. tetanic.

11. In caring for a client who has had a subtotal thyroidectomy, the nurse should assess for which immediate life-threatening complication?
    A. Hemorrhage
    B. Tetany
    C. Dehydration
    D. Laryngeal nerve damage

12. When collecting data on a client suspected of having an endocrine disorder, the nurse should observe for which sign?
    A. Kernig's sign
    B. Turner's sign
    C. Cushing's sign
    D. Trousseau's sign

13. What diagnostic test should the nurse anticipate for pancreas function?
    A. Cortisol
    B. Growth hormone
    C. Fasting blood glucose
    D. Ketones

14. Which of the following are the chemical messengers of the body?
    A. Hormones
    B. Thyroids
    C. Medullas
    D. Pituitaries

15. The creation of new glucose is called:
    A. glycogenolysis
    B. gluconeogenesis
    C. hyperglycemia
    D. hypoglycemia

Chapter 35

Caring for Clients With Endocrine Disorders

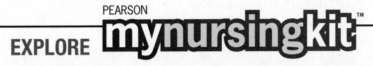

EXPLORE PEARSON **mynursingkit™**

MyNursingKit is your one stop for online chapter review materials and resources. Prepare for success with additional NCLEX®-style practice questions, interactive assignments and activities, web links, animations and videos, and more!

Register your access code from the front of your book at
www.mynursingkit.com

KEY TERMS

Match each term with its appropriate definition.

✓ D 1. SIADH	A. Results from adrenocorticotropic hormone insufficiency
✓ E 2. Dwarfism	B. Stimulates the hypersecretion of growth hormone that causes acromegaly
✓ B 3. Pituitary adenoma	C. Concentration of particles in the blood
G 4. Hyperthyroidism	D. Caused by an excess production of antidiuretic hormone
H 5. Diabetes insipidus	E. Caused by inadequate production of growth hormone
✓ F 6. Graves' disease	F. Hyperthyroidism
A 7. Addison's disease	G. Excessive production of thyroid hormone
C 8. Osmolarity	H. Insufficient amounts of adrenal cortex hormones
✓ J 9. Tetany	I. Common cause of primary hypothyroidism
I 10. Thyroiditis	J. Occurs with reduced calcium in the blood

LEARNING OUTCOMES

1. Define diabetes insipidus.

2. Describe a thyrotoxic crisis.

3. Describe a goiter.

4. Identify manifestations associated with myxedema coma.

5. Define tetany.

6. Describe Cushing's syndrome.

7. Identify symptoms associated with Addison's disease.

8. Identify nursing diagnoses regarding endocrine disorders.

9. Define pheochromocytoma.

10. Identify medications used for Addison's disease.

APPLY WHAT YOU LEARNED

You are caring for a client who presented to the emergency room with extreme fatigue, weight gain of more than 10 pounds in the last month, decreased appetite, slurred speech, and a puffy face. The client tells you that she is always cold and can not seem to warm up.

1. What diagnostic tests would the nurse expect to see ordered by the physician?

2. According to the symptoms listed above, is this a case of hyper- or hypothyroidism?

3. What medications and other treatments would the nurse expect to see?

MULTIPLE CHOICE

Circle the answer that best completes the following statements.

1. A client, diagnosed with acromegaly, tells you that he is having increased difficulty walking up the stairs at his house. Based on this statement, the nurse prepares a care plan for a nursing diagnosis of:
    A. Disturbed Body Image related to physical changes.
    B. Activity Intolerance related to joint pain.
    C. Pain related to increased weight on joints.
    D. Risk for Injury.

2. Mrs. Kay presents with a temperature of 101°F, malaise, and decreased lung sounds. She has a prescription for L-thyroxine, but tells you that she cannot afford the medication. During the assessment, she rapidly progresses to confusion and subsequently becomes unresponsive. You suspect that Mrs. Kay will be diagnosed with:
    A. thyroiditis.
    B. severe bronchitis.
    C. myxedema.
    D. sepsis.

3. A client with a blood pressure of 210/160, severe headaches, diaphoresis, tachycardia, and flushed skin is most likely suffering from:
    A. thyroid crisis.
    B. pheochromocytoma.
    C. goiter.
    D. Cushing's syndrome.

4. The nursing intervention that has the highest priority for the client who has undergone a subtotal thyroidectomy should be:
   A. assess for hemorrhage.
   B. assess for absent bowel sounds.
   C. assess for calcium deficiency.
   D. assess for laryngeal nerve damage.

5. An elderly woman with hyperparathyroidism is also likely to have:
   A. hypophosphatemia.
   B. hyponatremia.
   C. hypercalcemia.
   D. osteomyelitis.

6. The first priority for treating hypoparathyroidism is to administer:
   A. 500 mL of normal saline.
   B. calcium gluconate.
   C. vitamin D.
   D. calciferol.

7. Treatment for the client with hypothyroidism is:
   A. 500 mL of normal saline.
   B. lifelong.
   C. vitamin D.
   D. short term.

8. Mr. Tracy was diagnosed with hyperthyroidism 15 years ago. Recently he has been experiencing difficulty breathing and swallowing. You suspect:
   A. thyroid cancer.
   B. hyperparathyroidism.
   C. hypocalcemia.
   D. stroke.

9. Mrs. Kim has been complaining of lower back pain for 6 months. Today her labs show elevated levels of serum calcium, PTH, and alkaline phosphatase. These manifestations confirm a diagnosis of:
   A. stroke.
   B. hypocalcemia.
   C. hyperparathyroidism.
   D. thyroid cancer.

10. Nursing care of the client with hypoparathyroidism must consider the client's risk for injury due to:
    A. falls.
    B. tetany.
    C. altered thought processes.
    D. impaired memory.

11. Hirsutism is also recognized as:
    A. excessive facial hair.
    B. loss of facial hair.
    C. balding.
    D. thyroid skin.

12. Cushing's syndrome is more common in women between the ages of:
    A. 15 and 30.
    B. 20 and 50.
    C. 25 and 40.
    D. 30 and 45.

13. Hypercalcemia may lead to kidney stones, which are also known as:
    A. calculi.
    B. boils.
    C. striations.
    D. cysts.

14. Nursing care for a client with hypothermia would include:
    A. applying cool compresses.
    B. using a window fan to circulate the air.
    C. avoiding drafts.
    D. removing blankets.

15. The term euthyroid is used to describe:
    A. balanced thyroid.
    B. hyperthyroidism.
    C. hypothyroidism.
    D. Graves' disease.

Chapter 36

Caring for Clients With Diabetes Mellitus

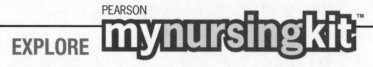

EXPLORE PEARSON mynursingkit™

MyNursingKit is your one stop for online chapter review materials and resources. Prepare for success with additional NCLEX®-style practice questions, interactive assignments and activities, web links, animations and videos, and more!

Register your access code from the front of your book at
www.mynursingkit.com

KEY TERMS

Match each term with its appropriate definition.

F _____ 1. Hyperglycemia   A. Condition of insufficient insulin production

H _____ 2. Type 1 diabetes   B. Chemical that regulates blood glucose levels

E _____ 3. Polydipsia   C. Morning rise of blood glucose after low levels at night

I _____ 4. Gangrene   D. Numbness or tingling in feet and hands

J _____ 5. Gluconeogenesis   E. Increased thirst

G _____ 6. Ketosis   F. High levels of circulating blood sugar

D _____ 7. Distal paresthesia   G. Toxic accumulation of ketone bodies

B _____ 8. Insulin   H. Requires insulin injections to sustain life

C _____ 9. Somogyi effect   I. Necrosis of tissue followed by infection

A _____ 10. Type 2 diabetes   J. Synthesis of glucose in the liver and kidneys

LEARNING OUTCOMES

1. Identify the key differences between type 1 and type 2 diabetes.

2. Describe the manifestations involved with type 1 diabetes.

3. Define glycosuria.

4. Identify the four types of insulin.

5. Describe the onset, peak, and duration of long-acting insulin.

6. Describe nursing implications for administering insulin.

7. Discuss nutritional recommendations for adults with diabetes.

8. Define ketonuria.

9. Identify characteristics of hyperosmolar hyperglycemia.

10. Describe clinical manifestations of peripheral vascular disease.

APPLY WHAT YOU LEARNED

A newly admitted client to your unit has had diabetes for 12 years. He is 64 years old and works third shift. He tells you that they order out a lot at work which usually consists of hamburgers, Chinese food, and pizza. When checking his blood glucose, the meter reads 312. Upon inspection of his skin, you notice that his feet have small sores developing bilaterally. The doctor is notified of these results and will be in to evaluate.

1. What dietary teaching could the nurse provide to this client?

2. What would the nurse expect regarding the treatment of a 312 glucose?

3. What hygiene teaching could the nurse provide in relation to the sores on the feet?

MULTIPLE CHOICE

Circle the answer that best completes the following statements.

1. The nurse understands that the diabetic client must be cautious when exercising because:
   A. blood sugar levels may drop rapidly.
   B. hyperglycemia may develop.
   C. insulin dosages need to be increased.
   D. exercise produces fatigue and weakness.

2. The nurse is explaining the action of an oral antidiabetic agent. The best statement that reflects the nurse's understanding is:
   A. the medication increases the production of natural insulin.
   B. beta cells are stimulated to release more insulin in response to hyperglycemia.
   C. oral agents provide long-acting release of previously injected pork insulin.
   D. antidiabetic agents slow insulin production by the pancreas.

3. Jacob is being evaluated for possible diabetes mellitus. When collecting the initial data, the nurse should ask:
   A. "Do you eat a lot of sweets?"
   B. "How long have you been overweight?"
   C. "Do you have to urinate frequently?"
   D. "Have you had this type of blood work done before?"

4. The nurse is discussing hypoglycemic reactions with a family. Which of the following statements made by the spouse indicates further teaching is not needed?
   A. "I'll make sure that we have some hard candy at home."
   B. "The coffee will make him wake up real fast."
   C. "His son is going to pick up some hamburgers for later."
   D. "We have some wine in the refrigerator if he gets too sleepy."

5. A newly diagnosed client with diabetes is concerned about his children. He asks if they should be tested for hyperglycemia. The correct nursing response is:
   A. "Probably; diabetes may be hereditary."
   B. "Yes, your children will have the same condition."
   C. "No, the disease is caused by a virus."
   D. "It's better to find out now than later."

6. A major characteristic found in insulin-dependent diabetes would include which of following?
   A. Generally resistant to the development of ketosis.
   B. Usually occurs before the age of 30.
   C. Pancreas produces small amount of insulin.
   D. Considered an autoimmune destruction of the alpha cells.

7. The nurse is teaching a class on the care of a diabetic client. She states that early signs of diabetic ketoacidosis are:
   A. cool, clammy skin and nervousness.
   B. hunger, headache, tremors.
   C. dark, scanty urine and diarrhea.
   D. thirst, dry mucous membranes and poor skin turgor.

8. A vial of insulin is labeled U-100. The nurse recognizes this as:
   A. 100 mg/unit.
   B. 100 units/bottle.
   C. 100 units/dose.
   D. 100 units/mL.

9. If the nurse needs to decide how soon before a meal to give an insulin injection, which of the following must be considered?
   A. Onset
   B. Peak
   C. Duration
   D. Limit

10. A diabetic client is seated in the waiting area of your clinic. He begins to complain of nausea and hunger. You observe that he is sweating, experiencing a few chills, and has cool, pale skin. You recognize that this client may be experiencing:
    A. hypotension.
    B. hyperglycemia.
    C. hypoglycemia.
    D. hypocalcemia.

11. Which of the following is the correct procedure for mixing insulins?
    A. Inject air into NPH vial, inject air into regular vial, withdraw regular insulin first.
    B. Inject air into regular vial, inject air into NPH vial, withdraw NPH first.
    C. Withdraw regular insulin first, then withdraw NPH.
    D. Withdraw NPH first, then withdraw regular insulin.

12. A client is admitted to the hospital, diagnosed with type 2 diabetes mellitus, and scheduled for discharge the following day. The nurse realizes that the short hospital stay is not sufficient for adequate diabetic teaching; therefore, the client's education should:
    A. include specific, realistic goals.
    B. reflect a complete care plan that can be implanted by the home health nurse.
    C. be concise, comprehensive, and intense.
    D. involve the client's family only.

13. Mr. Jackson, diagnosed with type 2 DM, is prescribed an 1800-calorie diet with daily exercise. The client's assessment data include: T-98.6, P-90, R-20, BP-160/98, height—5'5", weight—185 pounds. A dietary counseling referral was requested. The primary goal of nutritional therapy is:
    A. control of dietary intake to achieve ideal body weight.
    B. elimination of simple sugars.
    C. reduction in dietary calories to maintain normal blood pressure.
    D. daily equal distribution of carbohydrates.

14. A client has been seen by the diabetes education nurse. You determine that additional teaching is necessary when the client says:
    A. "I may have an occasional beer if I include it in my meal plan."
    B. "I will need a bedtime snack."
    C. "I can eat as much as I want to as long as I cover it with additional insulin."
    D. "I should eat my meals, even if I am not hungry."

15. A 16-year-old male client has been using self-capillary blood glucose monitoring as part of his diabetic management. After evaluating his technique, the nurse identifies a need for additional teaching because the client:
    A. chose a puncture site in the center of the finger pad.
    B. washed his hands before the procedure.
    C. told the nurse that 110 mg/dL is a well-controlled value.
    D. disposes of the lancet in a sharps container.

Chapter 37

The Nervous System and Assessment

KEY TERMS

Match each term with its appropriate definition.

_____ 1. CNS

_____ 2. PNS

_____ 3. Neuron

_____ 4. Axon

_____ 5. Myelin sheath

_____ 6. Synapse

_____ 7. Afferent neurons

_____ 8. Efferent neurons

_____ 9. Dermatome

_____ 10. ANS

A. An area of skin supplied by a single spinal nerve

B. Basic cell of the nervous system

C. Carries impulses away from the cell body

D. The cranial nerves, the spinal nerves, and the autonomic nervous system

E. The brain and spinal cord

F. System responsible for maintaining the body's internal homeostasis

G. A white, fatty substance that protects and insulates axons

H. Carry impulses from the skin and muscles to the CNS

I. Carry impulses from the CNS to the muscles and glands

J. A junction between neurons

LEARNING OUTCOMES

1. Define myelin sheath.

2. Identify the three layers of meninges.

3. Describe the cerebellum.

4. Define reflex.

5. Discuss the autonomic nervous system.

6. Describe Cheyne–Stokes.

7. Identify age-related changes in vision.

8. Define dysphagia.

9. Name the tenth cranial nerve, and describe its functions.

10. Define neurotransmitter.

APPLY WHAT YOU LEARNED

The student nurse is studying the topic of the nervous system this semester. He understands that there are different portions of the brain that have their own action and responsibility to the body. He also understands that there are 12 cranial nerves that play a role in the nervous system and control certain functions as well.

1. What cranial nerves are involved with difficulty swallowing?

2. What cranial nerves are related to eyeball movement?

MULTIPLE CHOICE

Circle the answer that best completes the following statements.

1. A number of changes in the eye and vision occur with aging. The lens becomes less elastic, affecting near vision. This is known as:
   A. myopia.
   B. nystagmus.
   C. irreversible hyperopia.
   D. presbyopia.

2. Normal cerebrospinal fluid contains:
   A. a few WBCs.
   B. a few RBCs.
   C. +3 protein.
   D. glucose of 75 mg/dL.

3. Jeff, the victim of a head injury, has recovered completely except for trouble speaking. What area of his brain was likely affected?
   A. Temporal lobe
   B. Broca's area
   C. Parietal lobe
   D. Wernicke's area

4. Mrs. Mave, 65, had a stroke. She is having difficulty understanding what you say or write to her. You suspect what area of her brain was affected?
   A. Broca's area
   B. Parietal lobe
   C. Wernicke's area
   D. Temporal lobe

5. A client with Bell's palsy most likely has involvement of what cranial nerve?
   A. VII
   B. X
   C. I
   D. XI

6. Loss of fat and subcutaneous tissue around the eyes generally leads to:
   A. difficulty focusing.
   B. reduced light entering the eye.
   C. decreased peripheral vision.
   D. increased risk of infection.

7. Ivan's parents complain of him zoning out for periods of time during the day. Ivan has no recollection of these times and sleeps heavily afterward. You suspect Ivan may have seizures. What test would determine if that diagnosis is correct?
   A. CT
   B. Myelography
   C. EMG
   D. MRI

8. Which test is used to detect brain cancer, Alzheimer's disease, epilepsy, and Parkinson's disease?
   A. EEG
   B. PET
   C. EMG
   D. CT

9. Tracy, an 18-year-old epileptic, is visibly upset when you enter her room. She is crying and states, "I can't get this gunk out of my hair!" You realize that she has just had a(n):
   A. MRI.
   B. EEG.
   C. PET.
   D. CT.

10. Mark has been complaining about his eye hurting ever since the car accident two days ago that broke his windshield. You suspect he may have glass in his eye. What type of test would confirm your suspicions?
    A. Visual field test
    B. CT
    C. Fluorescein stain
    D. MRI

11. A neuron is composed of all of the following except:
    A. dendrites.
    B. cell bodies.
    C. axons.
    D. nephrons.

12. The brain receives about how many mL of blood each minute?
    A. 750 mL
    B. 500 mL
    C. 1500 mL
    D. 250 mL

13. The nurse knows that there are how many pairs of cervical nerves?
    A. 8
    B. 12
    C. 5
    D. 10

14. What is the term used for eyelid drooping?
    A. Nystagmus
    B. Ptosis
    C. Dysphagia
    D. Presbyopia

15. In assessing for hearing difficulty, the nurse will ask about tinnitus, which is:
    A. need for increased volume.
    B. ringing in the ears.
    C. need for decreased volume.
    D. wax buildup in the ear.

Chapter 38

Caring for Clients With Intracranial Disorders

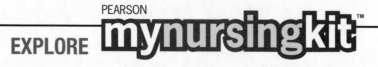

EXPLORE PEARSON **mynursingkit**

MyNursingKit is your one stop for online chapter review materials and resources. Prepare for success with additional NCLEX®-style practice questions, interactive assignments and activities, web links, animations and videos, and more!

Register your access code from the front of your book at
www.mynursingkit.com

KEY TERMS

Match each term with its appropriate definition.

_____ 1. TBI

_____ 2. Otorrhea

_____ 3. Battle's sign

_____ 4. ICP

_____ 5. Obtundation

_____ 6. CVA

_____ 7. TIA

_____ 8. Aneurysm

_____ 9. Seizure

_____ 10. Status epilepticus

A. A brief episode of reversible neurologic deficits

B. Pressure exerted within the cranium by the brain, blood, and CSF

C. A brain attack

D. A brief disruption of brain function caused by abnormal electrical activity in the nerve cells of the brain

E. State in which client responds to verbal and tactile stimuli but quickly drifts back to sleep

F. A life-threatening medical emergency that can cause permanent brain damage

G. An abnormal dilation of a cerebral artery

H. A leading cause of death and disability in the United States

I. Bruising over the mastoid process

J. CSF leaks from the ears

LEARNING OUTCOMES

1. Define hematoma.

2. Identify manifestations of a concussion.

3. Identify the three types of hematomas.

4. Describe altered level of consciousness.

5. Define brain tumors.

6. Identify manifestations related to brain tumors.

7. Define cerebrovascular accident.

8. Describe a seizure.

9. Define status epilepticus.

10. Describe meningitis.

APPLY WHAT YOU LEARNED

You are working the triage department in the ER when a client comes to you and tells you that he cannot feel his left arm or leg, has double vision, slight facial droop, and trouble finding the "right" words. The client has no known allergies that he is aware of and denies chest pain.

1. Based upon the manifestations above, what could be the diagnosis?

2. What diagnostic tests would the nurse expect to be ordered?

3. What is the treatment plan that the nurse will implement in this situation?

MULTIPLE CHOICE

Circle the answer that best completes the following statements.

1. Why is death a concern when discussing a client who has developed cerebral edema?
   A. There is decreased fluid to the brain, which causes dehydration.
   B. The force of the excess fluid may cause the brain to herniate.
   C. It is irreversible.
   D. If the edema lasts longer than 24 hours, death is inevitable.

2. You obtain the following results of a client's neurologic assessment: eyes open on command, disjointed conversation ability, unable to answer questions appropriately or to follow instructions. Based on the Glasgow Coma scale this client should be placed at:
   A. 9.
   B. 11.
   C. 15.
   D. 18.

3. Andrew Smythe has been diagnosed with a CVA due to an embolism. He has global aphasia and requires moderate assistance with ADL. Which of the following would not be an appropriate nursing diagnosis for Mr. Smythe?
   A. Ineffective Tissue Perfusion
   B. Self-Care Deficit
   C. Communication: Verbal, Impaired
   D. Urinary Incontinence, Total

4. Tejas has developed increased intracranial pressure due to an infection. You know to monitor for signs and symptoms of cerebral anoxia because:
   A. infections cause a decrease in blood flow to the brain.
   B. increased ICP creates an increased blood flow to the damaged area.
   C. increased ICP may prevent adequate blood flow to the brain.
   D. cerebral anoxia is a symptom of decreased ICP.

5. Jenny is a 2-year-old child diagnosed with a brain tumor. Which of the following questions would be appropriate to ask the child's mother?
   A. "Has Jenny been having trouble staying awake?"
   B. "Does Jenny have any problems with nausea?"
   C. "Have you noticed any changes in Jenny's speech?"
   D. All of the above questions would be appropriate.

6. Malcolm suffered a head injury after a motorcycle crash. The doctor explains that after a head injury it is not uncommon for a client to have one or two seizures. If the seizures occur in a chronic pattern, then the client will likely be diagnosed as having:
   A. adult-onset seizure disorder.
   B. convulsion disorder.
   C. epilepsy.
   D. seizures.

7. Malcolm has been given a new order for phenytoin 100 mg P.O. b.i.d. You are providing teaching about this medication. What information would you not include?
   A. Driving a vehicle is permitted after the first dose.
   B. CNS or vision changes must be reported to the doctor immediately.
   C. Take the medication with food or after meals.
   D. Blood levels should be checked on a routine basis.

8. Stephanie is a 33-year-old female who developed meningitis after a sinus infection. She has not responded well to the antibiotics and steroids. She asks if she will return to normal after the infection has cleared up. Your best response would be:
   A. "You should recover without complications."
   B. "There is a risk for long-term problems, such as vision or hearing changes."
   C. "Let me call the doctor so he can explain your prognosis to you."
   D. "You will likely be blind and deaf if you recover."

9. Mrs. Deib is 12 hours status postcraniotomy. Which of the following should be included on her nursing care plan?
   A. Keep the head of the bed at 90 degrees.
   B. Encourage Mrs. Deib to eat her prunes every morning.
   C. Obtain vital signs every 8 hours.
   D. Avoid sneezing and straining during bowel movements.

10. Heather is suspected of having a brain tumor. She has become impulsive and has difficulty making decisions. You suspect that her tumor is located in the:
    A. temporal lobe.
    B. frontal lobe.
    C. occipital lobe.
    D. parietal lobe.

11. During the assessment of a client experiencing headaches, the client tells the nurse that she has had headaches off and on during the past several years. She also says that she becomes severely nauseated when the pain of the

headache begins. Her only management for these headaches has been sleep. The nurse suspects she has:

A. migraine headaches.
B. tension headaches.
C. cluster headaches.
D. general headaches.

12. The first priority when a client begins to have a grand mal seizure should be to:

A. time the length of the seizure.
B. administer Valium to stop the seizure.
C. place a tongue depressor in the mouth.
D. maintain an open airway without restricting the client's movements.

13. Altered level of consciousness is likely to be observed in a client with:

A. increased ICP.
B. strokes, head injury, or meningitis.
C. any injury that causes a decrease of oxygen or glucose to the brain.
D. injuries that primarily affect the cranial nerves.

14. Which of the following interventions would be appropriate for any intracranial disorder?

A. Bowel management, diuretics, anticoagulants
B. Fall prevention, ADL assistance, bowel management
C. Anticoagulants, fall prevention, ADL assistance
D. Reorientation, caregiver training, fall prevention

15. A client has lost his ability to chew because of a stroke. The nurse knows that the nerve of mastication is called the:

A. vagus.
B. abducens.
C. trigeminal.
D. trochlear.

Chapter 39

Caring for Clients With Degenerative Neurologic and Spinal Cord Disorders

KEY TERMS

Match each term with its appropriate definition.

_____ 1. Rhizotomy

_____ 2. Dopamine

_____ 3. Bradykinesia

_____ 4. Sundowning

_____ 5. Chorea

_____ 6. Thymectomy

_____ 7. Fasciculations

_____ 8. Demyelination

_____ 9. Sciatica

_____ 10. Myelography

A. Involuntary contraction of skeletal muscles

B. Destruction or loss of myelin sheath

C. Visualization of spinal cord using x-rays

D. Surgical severing of a nerve root

E. Slowed speech or movement

F. Pain that follows the sciatic nerve

G. Surgical removal of the thymus gland

H. Uncontrollable, jerky movements

I. Increased confusion in evening or late hours

J. Neurotransmitter that inhibits voluntary motor function

LEARNING OUTCOMES

1. Define Alzheimer's disease.

2. Describe sundowning syndrome.

3. Describe the purpose of plasmapheresis.

4. Identify manifestations related to Parkinson's disease.

5. Define Huntington's disease.

6. Describe ALS.

7. Define rabies.

8. Discuss spinal cord injuries.

9. Define autonomic dysreflexia.

10. Describe spinal cord tumors.

APPLY WHAT YOU LEARNED

The student nurse is learning about neurologic disorders. Nursing diagnoses related to multiple sclerosis focus on coping, deficits in self-care, and continuing care. The student nurse is trying to understand this disorder in order to educate a client the nurse has seen on clinical rotations.

1. What topics would the student nurse discuss with the client and family to better understand the disorder?

2. What could the student nurse suggest regarding coping issues?

MULTIPLE CHOICE

Circle the answer that best completes the following statements.

1. Rodney is recovering from a fracture of the T3–T5 vertebra after a fall. He has made significant progress in rehabilitation and is due to be discharged home. The primary nursing diagnosis for his discharge planning will be:
   A. Risk for Autonomic Dysreflexia.
   B. Risk for Impaired Skin Integrity.
   C. Ineffective Individual Coping.
   D. Self-Care Deficit: Toileting.

2. The primary nursing intervention for a client with a newly placed Halo vest is:
   A. cleansing the pin sites every four hours.
   B. inspecting the pins and traction bars for tightness.
   C. turning the client every two hours.
   D. providing pain relief as needed.

3. Angus is 24 hours status postspinal fusion of L1–L2. Which of the following should be documented on the nursing care plan?
   A. Remove collar during the dressing change.
   B. Ensure the corset is applied correctly.
   C. Assess the donor site at the iliac crest.
   D. Assess the client for LOC, headache, and blurred vision.

4. You are preparing a client for a myelography. The client needs further teaching if he states:
   A. "After the test, I should drink lots of fluids."
   B. "The dye is going to make me feel a bit cool."
   C. "I won't drink anything for several hours before the test."
   D. "I will definitely try to void as soon as I feel the urge."

5. A client diagnosed with multiple sclerosis is being prepared for discharge. The nurse is assessing the client's home care. The most important question to ask the client is:
   A. "Do you understand the disease process for MS?"
   B. "Will you be able to prepare a well-balanced meal?"
   C. "Do you have enough financial resources to help you through this crisis?"
   D. "Is there anyone at home who has a cold?"

6. A 32-year-old woman presents to the emergency room and is diagnosed by the doctor with a cholinergic crisis. Which of the following represents the most appropriate question in order to gain information about this condition?
   A. "Do you feel short of breath?"
   B. "How much of the neostigmine did you take this week?"
   C. "Have you had any nausea or vomiting?"
   D. "Have you experienced any fast heartbeats?"

7. A mother asks the nurse if her child really needs to receive a tetanus vaccine or if there is some other preventive measure that would be more effective. The best response should be:
   A. "He needs the vaccine."
   B. "The vaccine will decrease his chances of developing tetanus."
   C. "If you clean all of his cuts right away, there really is no need for the injection."
   D. "You won't have to worry anymore about tetanus if he gets the shot."

8. Mr. Jones has been taking Haldol for the treatment of a mild psychosis. He displays a shuffling gait, mild hand tremors, and slurred speech. The nurse knows that these symptoms may be clinical manifestations of:
   A. Parkinson's disease.
   B. parkinsonism.
   C. Tourette's syndrome.
   D. Creutzfeldt–Jakob disease.

9. The primary nursing intervention during the assessment of a person with a spinal cord injury is to:
   A. ensure that the person's head remains immobile.
   B. assess the respiratory status.
   C. maintain the airway.
   D. assess for autonomic dysreflexia.

10. Douglas was in a car crash several weeks ago and has now been admitted to the rehabilitation facility for further evaluation of his T3 injury. During his teaching session, the nurse should remind Douglas to:
    A. call the nurse for any severe headache.
    B. report a rise in his blood pressure.
    C. report the sensation of a full bladder.
    D. ask for help when ambulating to the bathroom.

11. Wanda has had a laminectomy two hours ago and is complaining of a headache. You logroll her to inspect the dressing on her back. There is a large amount of clear drainage noted on the gauze. Your next action should be to:
    A. remove the dressing to check the incision site.
    B. raise the head of the bed to relieve the headache.
    C. test the drainage with a glucose reagent strip.
    D. call the doctor.

12. An elderly client, admitted for a hernia repair, has become confused and agitated during the evening shift. The nurse suspects that the client is suffering from sundowning. Which of the following actions is appropriate for this client?
    A. Restrain the client's hands.
    B. Close the door so he won't disturb the other clients.
    C. Document the behavior.
    D. Ask a nursing assistant to stay in the room until a plan of care is formulated.

13. The most effective drug for the treatment of Parkinson's disease is:
    A. Sinemet.
    B. Parlodel.
    C. Permax.
    D. levodopa.

14. A client with severe muscle spasms from a spinal cord injury calls the nurse for any medication that will decrease the pain. The nurse checks the doctor's orders and administers:
    A. diazepam.
    B. Tensilon.
    C. Artane.
    D. Cogentin.

15. Sarah has a complete spinal cord injury at the level of T1. She develops spinal shock. Which of the following are manifestations of this condition?
    A. Tachycardia
    B. Hypertension
    C. Diaphoresis
    D. Flaccid paralysis

Chapter 40

Caring for Clients With Eye and Ear Disorders

KEY TERMS

Match each term with its appropriate definition.

_____ 1. Conjunctiva

_____ 2. Depth perception

_____ 3. Iris

_____ 4. Tympanic membrane

_____ 5. Hearing

_____ 6. Pinna

_____ 7. Cerumen

_____ 8. Lacrimal gland

_____ 9. Macula

_____ 10. Pupil

A. Membrane that lines the anterior surface of the eye

B. Perception and interpretation of sound

C. Area of central vision in the retina

D. Produces tears to moisten and irrigate the eye

E. Vibrates and transmits sound to the middle ear

F. Earwax

G. Controls the amount of light that enters the eye

H. Ability to identify distances between objects

I. Colored portion of the eye

J. External portion of the ear

LEARNING OUTCOMES

1. Define conjunctivitis.

2. Describe cataracts.

3. Identify manifestations regarding glaucoma.

4. Discuss the assessment of visual fields by confrontation.

5. Define retinal detachments.

6. Describe macular degeneration.

7. Identify tips to prevent external otitis.

8. Define tinnitus.

9. Describe vertigo.

10. Identify nursing diagnoses related to hearing loss.

APPLY WHAT YOU LEARNED

A 55-year-old male presents to your clinic for a follow-up regarding his blindness. He had a chemical exposure accident one month ago and has been trying to adapt to his new lifestyle. His wife and teenage son are very supportive and have modified the house to better assist with his independence.

1. How can the nurse help foster independence with this client?

2. How can the family ensure adequate nutrition?

3. What services would be appropriate for this client?

MULTIPLE CHOICE

Circle the answer that best completes the following statements.

1. The nurse is preparing a discharge instruction sheet for a client who had ear surgery two days ago. Which of the following must be included in this plan?
   A. Take antiemetics t.i.d.
   B. Change the inner dressing daily.
   C. Keep the mouth open when sneezing or coughing.
   D. Do not bathe until released by the doctor.

2. A client with newly diagnosed glaucoma is receiving eyedrops for the first time. After instilling the drops you gently squeeze the bridge of his nose for 1 minute. He asks you why you are pinching his nose. The best response should be:
   A. "If I pinch the nose, you won't move around as much."
   B. "It keeps more of the medication in your eye."
   C. "Pinching the nose increases the blood supply to the eyes."
   D. "I'm sorry. I shouldn't have pinched your nose for such a long time."

3. You are responding to an accident in the hospital kitchen. A coworker is bleeding from her right eye. Upon examination you see a small shard of metal penetrating her eye through the eyelid. Your next action is to:
   A. irrigate the eye with normal saline.
   B. remove the object, then irrigate the eye.
   C. place a cup over the injured eye and tell her to keep the other eye closed.
   D. take her to the emergency room.

4. A cataract is:
   A. a clouding of the eye lens.
   B. the filling of the space between the lens and cornea with aqueous humor.
   C. an occluded canal of Schlemm.
   D. incurable and leads to blindness.

5. After eye surgery, a client is instructed not to bend over for a couple of days because:
   A. eye pressure increases when bending at the waist.
   B. the medication will flow out of the eye.
   C. it may cause shooting pains in the eye.
   D. the bending movement will increase the pain.

6. A client with glaucoma asks how long he must use eyedrops. The nurse responds:
   A. "Sorry, for the rest of your life."
   B. "When the canal of Schlemm opens completely and remains open."
   C. "It all depends on the success of your surgery."
   D. "There is no way to correct your problem, so you must use the drops for life."

7. Xia Zihuen is a native Chinese woman with a diagnosis of retinal detachment. You are giving preoperative instructions regarding the corrective surgery. You should first:
   A. provide information about the mydriatic eyedrops.
   B. discuss the types of corrective lens available.
   C. explain that perfect vision may not be possible after the procedure.
   D. assess her language skills and educational level.

8. A young child is more likely to suffer from otitis media than an adult because:
   A. children are more susceptible to inner ear infections.
   B. the eustachian tube is more horizontal in children.
   C. children are more likely to get colds and flu.
   D. it is a common childhood illness.

9. The primary nursing diagnosis for a client experiencing an acute attack of vertigo is:
   A. Anxiety.
   B. Risk for Aspiration.
   C. Risk for Injury.
   D. Powerlessness.

10. You are teaching a client the proper positioning of the head for instilling eardrops in his right ear. The correct procedure would be to:
    A. lie on the affected side.
    B. tilt the head backward.
    C. tilt the head toward the unaffected side.
    D. tilt the head forward.

11. Which of the following is least likely to develop sensorineural hearing loss?
    A. Client with Meniere's disease
    B. Client with a perforated eardrum
    C. Construction worker
    D. Client on high doses of antibiotics

12. The nurse instructs a client who is using Betoptic eyedrops to check her pulse one hour after instillation of the medication. The rationale for this is:
    A. tachycardia is a severe side effect.
    B. the medication is a beta-blocker.
    C. Betoptic is contraindicated in COPD and heart failure patients.
    D. the doctor wants a report on the adverse reactions experienced by the client.

13. The nurse is conducting a Weber test on a 24-year-old client. He knows that the test is negative if the client hears:
    A. sound in both ears equally.
    B. sound in the right ear only.
    C. sound in the left ear only.
    D. no sound.

14. Which of the following is most likely to develop external otitis?
    A. Olympic swimmer
    B. Football player
    C. Karate teacher
    D. Hairdresser

15. The nurse is demonstrating the assessment of the six cardinal fields of vision in a continuing education class. A student asks, "What is the purpose of this test?" The nurse should state that the purpose is to:
    A. determine if the client has vision in those areas of the eye.
    B. determine if the client is able to follow directions.
    C. assess the smoothness of the eye movement.
    D. assess the function of the extraocular muscles.

Chapter 41

The Musculoskeletal System and Assessment

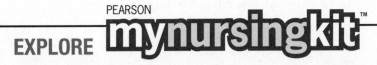

EXPLORE PEARSON **mynursingkit™**

MyNursingKit is your one stop for online chapter review materials and resources. Prepare for success with additional NCLEX®-style practice questions, interactive assignments and activities, web links, animations and videos, and more!

Register your access code from the front of your book at www.mynursingkit.com

KEY TERMS

Match each term with its appropriate definition.

_____ 1. Osteocytes   A. Manufactures blood cells and hemoglobin

_____ 2. Tendons   B. Cushions and protects bony areas

_____ 3. Skeletal muscle   C. Cells that are associated with resorption of bone

_____ 4. Yellow bone marrow   D. Provides involuntary movement

_____ 5. Bursae   E. Connects muscles to bone

_____ 6. Osteoblasts   F. Cells responsible for bone maintenance

_____ 7. Red bone marrow   G. Connects bones to bones

_____ 8. Smooth muscle   H. Cells associated with bone production

_____ 9. Ligaments   I. Contains fat and connective tissue

_____ 10. Osteoclasts   J. Allows voluntary movement

LEARNING OUTCOMES

1. Define ligaments.

2. Identify the three types of muscle tissue.

3. Describe abduction and adduction.

4. Describe ballottement.

5. Identify the purpose of an ESR.

6. Describe calcium testing related to musculoskeletal disorders.

7. Define bone densitometry.

8. Describe arthroscopy.

9. Define arthrocentesis.

10. Identify normal phosphate levels.

APPLY WHAT YOU LEARNED

A 52-year-old female presents to her physician with complaints of right knee pain that began about one week ago. She was gardening when it happened and it is not the result of a fall. She states that she was kneeling on it for about an hour and it is swollen and warm to the touch.

1. What diagnostic testing would the nurse expect to see ordered by the physician?

2. Would this client be appropriate for surgery? If so, which type?

MULTIPLE CHOICE

Circle the answer that best completes the following statements.

1. When caring for a client with a leg cast, which of these assessments requires immediate nursing intervention?
   A. Cool distal appendages
   B. Edematous foot
   C. Increased capillary refill
   D. Pain at 6 on a scale of 0 to 10

2. A client has sustained several rib fractures from falling off a roof. If all of these interventions are possible, which should have the highest priority?
   A. Administer analgesics as ordered.
   B. Encourage use of incentive spirometer.
   C. Splint chest for breathing or coughing.
   D. Assess respiratory status every four hours.

3. A nurse teaches a client how to care for a sprained ankle. Which of these statements indicates that further teaching is necessary?
   A. "I will keep my leg elevated as much as possible."
   B. "My prescription for my pain medication has been sent to the pharmacy."
   C. "I'm going to use a heating pad this evening."
   D. "My ace bandage is comfortable now."

4. You are assisting the nurse educator in teaching a class on proper range-of-motion techniques. She asks you to demonstrate the movement of pronation. You should:
   A. move in a circle.
   B. turn your palms down.
   C. bend your ankle upward.
   D. turn your foot outward.

5. Which of these nursing interventions is the most important when caring for a client with a fractured tibia?
   A. Neurovascular assessment
   B. Administering pain medications
   C. Respiratory assessment
   D. Cast care

6. Mrs. Dawson states that she is unable to complete normal daily activities because of the pain from her fibromyalgia. The most appropriate response by the nurse is:
   A. "I can ask the doctor to refer you to a psychiatrist for help."
   B. "Do you think the pain is real?"
   C. "I understand that this is painful. Exercise can be helpful."
   D. "You can't continue to depend on drugs to help you."

7. Which of the following behaviors observed by the nurse requires intervention to decrease the risk of back injury?
   A. The client care technician bends his knees to retrieve the client's slippers.
   B. The nursing assistant is pulling a large equipment cart down the hallway.
   C. A coworker uses a ladder to replace supplies on a top shelf.
   D. A nurse raises the bed to waist height to turn a client.

8. The nurse is instructing a client and his wife about a bone scan procedure scheduled for the afternoon. Which of the following should be discussed during this session?
   A. NPO status 8 hours before the procedure.
   B. Client will have to drink 8 ounces of contrast medium.
   C. The scan will take at least 30 to 60 minutes to complete.
   D. Radioactive precautions must be taken after the procedure.

9. Maintaining an active lifestyle and performing specific exercises such as weight training are two ways to help counteract aging changes, maintain muscle mass, and prevent:
   A. rheumatoid arthritis.
   B. osteoporosis.
   C. fractures.
   D. myeloma.

10. Ken complains of "water on the knee." What two assessments can you do to determine if he actually has extra fluid in his knee joint?
    A. Bulge sign and ballottement
    B. Thomas test and bulge sign
    C. Ballottement and Thomas test
    D. Arthrocentesis and bulge sign

11. Long bones of the skeleton have two broad ends known as:
    A. diaphysis.
    B. epiphyses.
    C. osteoblasts.
    D. periosteums.

12. The nurse understands that when a joint is bent at the limb, it is:
    A. flexed.
    B. extended.
    C. abducted.
    D. adducted.

13. In understanding muscle strength, a grade of 2 describes:
    A. full ROM against gravity.
    B. passive ROM.
    C. paralysis.
    D. full ROM against full resistance.

14. When a hip flexion contracture is suspected, which test should be performed?
    A. Ballottement test
    B. Kernig's sign
    C. Thomas test
    D. Bulge sign

15. When evaluating the toes, flexion means to:
    A. curl your toes.
    B. spread your toes.
    C. remain still.
    D. stand on your toes.

Chapter 42

Caring for Clients With Musculoskeletal Trauma

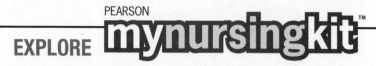

EXPLORE

MyNursingKit is your one stop for online chapter review materials and resources. Prepare for success with additional NCLEX®-style practice questions, interactive assignments and activities, web links, animations and videos, and more!

Register your access code from the front of your book at **www.mynursingkit.com**

KEY TERMS

Match each term with its appropriate definition.

_____ 1. Trauma

_____ 2. Contusion

_____ 3. Sprain

_____ 4. Strain

_____ 5. Fracture

_____ 6. Compartment syndrome

_____ 7. Reduction

_____ 8. Cast

_____ 9. Traction

_____ 10. Gangrene

A. Event that occurs when bone is subjected to more force than it can absorb

B. A rigid device used to immobilize broken bones and promote healing

C. Bleeding into soft tissue resulting from blunt force

D. Tissue death that can lead to amputation

E. Use of a straightening or pulling force to return or maintain the fractured bones in normal position

F. Restoration of normal alignment

G. A ligament injury

H. Excess pressure that restricts blood vessels and nerves

I. A microscopic tear in the muscle that causes bleeding into the tissues

J. Event that occurs when tissues are subjected to more force than they are able to absorb

LEARNING OUTCOMES

1. Identify characteristics of a sprain.

2. Define a fracture.

3. Describe compartment syndrome.

4. Define carpal tunnel syndrome.

5. Describe phantom pain.

6. Identify ways to decrease fractures in older adults.

7. Define traction.

8. Identify manifestations of compartment syndrome.

9. Describe a fat emboli.

10. Describe RICE.

APPLY WHAT YOU LEARNED

A 45-year-old male was admitted for a BKA related to gangrene as a consequence of his diabetes. He lives alone in a two-story home. He is angry as evidenced by shouting at all staff who try to assist him.

1. What nursing interventions relate to this situation?

2. How can the nurse assist this client with discharge planning?

MULTIPLE CHOICE

Circle the answer that best completes the following statements.

1. A client is admitted to the hospital with a fractured hip. Which of these statements describes the main goal of therapy?
   A. Alleviating pain
   B. Maintaining circulation
   C. Preventing additional trauma
   D. Increasing mobility

2. The nurse is discussing discharge instructions with a client who has undergone a below-the-knee amputation. Which action by the client would indicate acceptance of the body part loss?
   A. Verbalizing understanding of the dressing change
   B. Touching the incision
   C. Asking questions related to pain medication
   D. Looking at the amputation site

3. A plaster of Paris cast was applied to your client's left arm several hours ago. You were asked to teach the client how to care for the cast. Which of the following statements would indicate that the client understood your instructions?
   A. "Could I borrow a hair dryer to speed the drying process?"
   B. "Wow, my arm is warm."
   C. "Guess I won't need a sling now that I have this cast."
   D. "Look at the indentations in this cast!"

4. The nurse is admitting a client in the emergency room who sustained an injury while playing soccer. Which of the following clinical manifestations might indicate that the client's shoulder is dislocated?
   A. Edema of the upper arm
   B. Pain radiating to the wrist
   C. Increased length of the affected arm
   D. Bruising in the scapula region

5. Jerry twists his right ankle, injuring several ligaments. This injury is classified as a:
   A. sprain.
   B. strain.
   C. contusion.
   D. fracture.

6. A client's wrist is edematous and painful as a result of a sports accident. Initial treatment should include:
   A. elevation and heat application.
   B. elevation and ice application.
   C. elevation and ACE® bandage only.
   D. elevation and a splint.

7. A fracture that involves protrusion of the bone through the skin is a(n):
   A. complete fracture.
   B. compound fracture.
   C. greenstick fracture.
   D. oblique fracture.

8. A client has skeletal traction to her left leg. Appropriate nursing action to assist in transporting the client to the x-ray department would be:
   A. maintain traction during transport.
   B. remove weights before transporting.
   C. place weights on the bed.
   D. secure the weights on the traction frame.

9. Mrs. Carson has had a right hip arthroplasty. A priority nursing intervention during the postoperative phase is to:
   A. maintain the hip in adduction.
   B. maintain the hip in abduction.
   C. maintain the Buck's traction.
   D. perform active ROM on the right leg.

10. A client has an above-the-knee amputation resulting from uncontrolled diabetes. The nurse should recognize that the purpose of using an elastic wrap on the stump is to:
    A. prevent pain.
    B. prevent hemorrhage.
    C. prevent edema.
    D. prevent infection.

11. When grading a sprain, Grade II would indicate:
    A. complete tearing of the ligament.
    B. overstretching with mild bleeding and inflammation.
    C. severe stretching and some tearing with inflammation.
    D. the bony attachment of the ligament is broken away.

12. What type of traction is done by physically pulling on the extremity?
    A. Manual
    B. Skeletal
    C. Skin
    D. Balanced

13. What is a partial separation of the bones of a joint called?
    A. Subluxation
    B. Internal rotation
    C. External rotation
    D. Extracapsular

14. Another term for tennis elbow is:
    A. carpal tunnel.
    B. epicondylitis.
    C. arthritis.
    D. bursitis.

15. Phantom pain is associated with which surgical procedure?
    A. Arthroscopy
    B. Biopsy
    C. Amputation
    D. Replacement

Chapter 43

Caring for Clients With Musculoskeletal Disorders

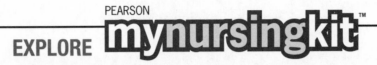

EXPLORE PEARSON mynursingkit™

MyNursingKit is your one stop for online chapter review materials and resources. Prepare for success with additional NCLEX®-style practice questions, interactive assignments and activities, web links, animations and videos, and more!

Register your access code from the front of your book at
www.mynursingkit.com

KEY TERMS

Match each term with its appropriate definition.

_____ 1. Ankylosing spondylitis   A. Loss of bone mass

_____ 2. Gout   B. Softening of the bones

_____ 3. Kyphosis   C. Bunion

_____ 4. Rheumatoid arthritis   D. Joint replacement

_____ 5. Arthroplasty   E. Chronic inflammation and stiffening of the spine

_____ 6. Scoliosis   F. Accumulation of uric acid crystals in the joints

_____ 7. Osteomalacia   G. Increased thoracic curvature

_____ 8. Hallux valgus   H. Systemic connective tissue inflammatory disorder

_____ 9. Osteoporosis   I. Lateral curvature of the spine

_____ 10. Arthralgia   J. Joint pain

LEARNING OUTCOMES

1. Define pathological fractures.

2. Identify risks for osteomyelitis.

3. Describe osteoarthritis.

4. Define rheumatoid arthritis.

5. Describe lupus.

6. Define fibromyalgia.

7. Describe muscular dystrophy.

8. Identify multisystem effects of lupus.

9. Identify manifestations of rheumatoid arthritis.

10. Define arthralgia.

APPLY WHAT YOU LEARNED

A 44-year-old male is currently in his second status post total knee replacement. He is preparing for discharge and is offering no complaints of pain, only minor discomfort with movement. He is scheduled for physical therapy as an outpatient. He resides on a first floor apartment with his wife.

1. Identify some teaching that the nurse will be doing with this client prior to discharge.

2. How can the nurse ensure that the client and his wife understand the discharge instructions?

MULTIPLE CHOICE

Circle the answer that best completes the following statements.

1. Mrs. Montez, age 58, is diagnosed with osteoporosis. The teaching plan should include which of the following points?
   A. Increase weight-bearing exercises.
   B. Increase isometric exercises.
   C. Reduce calcium intake.
   D. Increase protein intake.

2. The nurse informs a client with osteoporosis that a new drug has been prescribed to inhibit bone resorption. Which of the following medications has this action?
   A. Sodium fluoride
   B. Calcium carbonate
   C. Estrogen
   D. Alendronate

3. Hanna is diagnosed with SLE. The nurse would be most alarmed if Hanna developed:
   A. painful joints.
   B. severe headaches.
   C. abnormal breath sounds.
   D. weight loss.

4. Hydroxychloroquine has been prescribed for a client with systemic lupus. Client teaching should include:
   A. have eye examinations every six months.
   B. avoid the use of NSAIDs.
   C. measure output every eight hours.
   D. document daily weights.

5. A client is prescribed a low-purine diet. The nurse recognizes the need for further teaching if he chooses which food for lunch?
   A. Chicken
   B. Milk
   C. Liver
   D. Corn

6. Your client has been given a prescription for allopurinol. He calls the clinic to report that a rash has developed on his chest and arms. The nurse's best response would be:
   A. "Don't worry, it will go away in a few days."
   B. "Please stop taking the medication."
   C. "Discontinue the drug and make an appointment with your doctor right away."
   D. "Finish taking the pills and then schedule a follow-up appointment."

7. You are teaching a client about a high-calcium diet. The client understands the instructions if he tells you that the best source of calcium would be:
   A. a seafood platter.
   B. broccoli casserole.
   C. tofu.
   D. whole milk.

8. The nurse is developing a care plan for a client with gout. The diagnosis is Acute Pain. Which of the following interventions should be included in the plan of care?
   A. Increase outdoor activity.
   B. Wrap foot with an ACE® bandage.
   C. Keep the foot warm by covering with a sheet.
   D. Administer analgesics as ordered.

9. Joan went on a vacation in the mountains. One month after her return, she developed malaise, fever, muscle pain, and an unusual skin lesion. You suspect that the doctor will treat Joan for:
   A. Rocky Mountain spotted fever.
   B. Lyme disease.
   C. rabies.
   D. malaria.

10. A client is diagnosed with the most common malignant bone tissue tumor of the long bones. Based on your knowledge of bone tumors, you suspect that the tumor will be classified as:
   A. multiple myeloma.
   B. Ewing's sarcoma.
   C. chondrosarcoma.
   D. osteosarcoma.

11. The nurse is reviewing a client's medical records and notes that the ESR is elevated and the rheumatoid factor is positive. Using this knowledge, the nurse believes that the doctor will make a diagnosis of:
   A. rheumatoid arthritis.
   B. ankylosing spondylitis.
   C. muscular dystrophy.
   D. Paget's disease.

12. Gold salt therapy is prescribed for a client with rheumatoid arthritis. The primary function of this medication is to:
    A. reduce pain.
    B. reduce joint deformities.
    C. reduce inflammation.
    D. reduce infection.

13. Scoliosis is usually diagnosed:
    A. as a teen.
    B. as an older adult.
    C. as a young adult.
    D. as an infant.

14. A pregnant woman is recommended to have a calcium intake of:
    A. 400 mg.
    B. 1,200–1,500 mg.
    C. 800–1,200 mg.
    D. 1,000 mg.

15. Foods high in calcium include all of the following except:
    A. milk.
    B. yogurt.
    C. cheese.
    D. oranges.

Chapter 44

The Integumentary System and Assessment

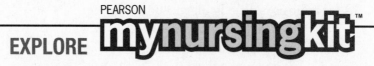

KEY TERMS

Match each term with its appropriate definition.

_____ 1. Melanin
_____ 2. Epidermis
_____ 3. Keratin
_____ 4. Dermis
_____ 5. Erythema
_____ 6. Vitiligo
_____ 7. Edema
_____ 8. Clubbing
_____ 9. Lentigines
_____ 10. Macule

A. Flat, nonpalpable change in skin color
B. Reddening of the skin
C. Angle of nail base is greater than 180 degrees
D. Outermost part of the skin, made of epithelial cells
E. Protects nerve endings in the dermis from the damaging effects of ultraviolet light
F. Hyperpigmentation called "liver spots"
G. An abnormal, patchy, loss of melanin, over the face, hands, and groin
H. A fibrous, water-repellent protein that makes the epidermis tough and protective
I. Deeper layer of skin made up of a flexible connective tissue
J. Accumulation of fluid in the body's tissues

LEARNING OUTCOMES

1. Define cyanosis.

2. Identify the function of the dermis.

3. Describe the three types of glands.

4. Describe a vesicle.

5. Discuss keloids.

6. Define clubbing.

7. Describe a biopsy.

8. Identify the purpose of a culture and sensitivity test regarding the skin.

9. Describe a patch test.

10. Define alopecia.

APPLY WHAT YOU LEARNED

The student nurse was instructed to receive a two-step PPD prior to starting clinical rotations. The student understands that this is a test to help identify the tuberculosis infection. The student also knows that it is done in steps over two weeks.

1. What physical sign would be present in a positive test?

MULTIPLE CHOICE

Circle the answer that best completes the following statements.

1. Caucasians have a pinkish skin tone because of:
   A. profuse erythema.
   B. blood leakage.
   C. red blood cells underneath skin.
   D. melanin.

2. The nurse is reviewing a client's record and notes that the medical history includes psoriasis. Based on her knowledge of this condition, the nurse does not expect to find which of the following clinical manifestations?
   A. Discoloration and pitting of the nailbeds
   B. Silvery-white scaly patches on the scalp, elbows, knees, and sacral area
   C. Gray areas of plaque
   D. Diffuse red rash

3. During inspection of a client's skin, the nurse observes an irregularly shaped, heavily pigmented "mole." The nurse's next action should be to:
   A. ask the client if he is aware of the mole.
   B. document the size, color, and appearance in the chart.
   C. notify the physician immediately.
   D. check the medical history in the records.

4. A teenager asks his nurse what is causing his acne. The nurse most appropriately responds by saying:
   A. "It's caused by eating lots of fried foods and chocolate."
   B. "It is caused by clogged oil glands."
   C. "The exact cause is not known."
   D. "It is caused by excessive sunlight and heat."

5. To soothe the itching of acne lesions, the nurse might suggest which of the following interventions?
   A. Cleanse lesions with soap and hot water.
   B. Teach the client to rub instead of scratching the lesions.
   C. Apply a soothing lotion to the face to relieve the itching.
   D. Rub the face briskly with a towel after cleansing.

6. A client is admitted to the neuro floor after experiencing a CVA with resulting left-sided paralysis. The most important nursing intervention at this time should be to:
   A. turn the client every two hours.
   B. place the client in a low-Fowler's position.
   C. limit fluid intake.
   D. consult with physical therapist to begin gait training.

7. Randy, 45, has been diagnosed with cirrhosis of the liver. He has a yellow pigment to his skin. You know this is called:
   A. jaundice.
   B. melaninic.
   C. keratotic.
   D. cyanotic.

8. You notice that your client's oxygen is not connected. His lips are starting to turn blue and he is lethargic. As you hook his oxygen back up and call the respiratory therapist, you realize his lips are:
   A. jaundiced.
   B. melanin.
   C. keratin.
   D. cyanotic.

9. You notice your neighbor, 57, outside in her garden. When you go outside to talk to her, she seems confused; thinking she may be dehydrated you check her skin for:
   A. bruising.
   B. rashes.
   C. erythema.
   D. tenting.

10. Red splinter hemorrhages and pigmented bands on nails are normal in 90% of:
    A. Caucasians.
    B. African Americans.
    C. Hispanics.
    D. Chinese.

11. Reddening of the skin is known as:
    A. erythema.
    B. cyanosis.
    C. blanching.
    D. necrosis.

12. The nurse knows that a client suffering from a liver disorder will appear:
    A. jaundiced.
    B. cyanotic.
    C. pallor.
    D. necrotic.

13. An insect bite or a hive will leave a mark known as a:
    A. nodule.
    B. pustule.
    C. wheal.
    D. macule.

14. The outermost part of the skin is:
    A. melanin.
    B. epidermis.
    C. dermis.
    D. glands.

15. Which gland secretes sebum?
    A. Apocrine
    B. Eccrine
    C. Sebaceous
    D. Thyroid

Chapter 45

Caring for Clients With Skin Disorders

KEY TERMS

Match each term with its appropriate definition.

_____ 1.	Pruritus	A.	Fever blister or cold sore
_____ 2.	Cellulitis	B.	Caused by the human papilloma virus
_____ 3.	Herpes zoster	C.	Infection at skin surface extending into hair follicle
_____ 4.	Acne	D.	Shingles
_____ 5.	Verrucae	E.	Athlete's foot
_____ 6.	Pediculosis	F.	Subjective itching sensation
_____ 7.	Exfoliative dermatitis	G.	Skin disorder of the sebaceous glands
_____ 8.	Herpes simplex	H.	Infestation with lice
_____ 9.	Tinea pedis	I.	Characterized by peeling skin
_____ 10.	Folliculitis	J.	Diffuse inflammation of the skin layers

LEARNING OUTCOMES

1. Define psoriasis.

2. Describe contact dermatitis.

3. Define cellulitis.

4. Describe folliculitis.

5. Define basal cell carcinoma.

6. Identify methods to prevent skin cancer.

7. Define pressure ulcers.

8. Identify the four stages in pressure ulcers.

9. Describe melanoma.

10. Define nevi.

APPLY WHAT YOU LEARNED

A 24-year-old female presents to the clinic with a growth on her nose. She states that she doesn't sun tan but opts for the tanning salon. She denies using any sunscreen or other protection while in the tanning bed. She is concerned about her appearance and does not believe the growth could be cancerous.

1. Describe the ABCD rule according to the American Cancer Society.

2. What type of cancer is this client manifesting?

3. What preventative measures can the nurse explain to this client?

MULTIPLE CHOICE

Circle the answer that best completes the following statements.

1. Mr. Williams is admitted to the hospital for treatment of acute cellulitis caused by a spider bite. He asks the nurse to explain what the term means. The nurse plans to base a response on the understanding that cellulitis is a(n):
   A. skin infection that extends into the subcutaneous tissue.
   B. acute superficial infection.
   C. inflammation of the epidermis.
   D. epidermal infection caused by staphylococcus.

2. The nurse is assessing a client and notices eczema on the back of his neck and bilateral knees. Based on her knowledge of this condition, the nurse expects to find:
   A. gray areas of plaque.
   B. a diffuse red rash.
   C. discoloration and pitting edema.
   D. silvery-white scaly patches.

3. The physician has just diagnosed a client with herpes simplex Type I. The nurse expects the medication ordered will be:
   A. triple antibiotic.
   B. Bactroban.
   C. acyclovir.
   D. actinex.

4. Retin-A is prescribed for the treatment of acne. The nurse questions the order if the medication is ordered for a:
   A. 12-year-old diagnosed with asthma.
   B. 15-year-old male diagnosed with cystic fibrosis.
   C. 20-year-old diagnosed with eczema.
   D. 25-year-old male diagnosed with HIV.

5. Marvin states he will not go the prom because of his acute acne. The most appropriate response by the nurse would be:
   A. "Lots of kids your age have zits. That's no reason to stay at home."
   B. "Can't you get a date?"
   C. "I can tell this upsets you. Please tell me more."
   D. "The lesions will be cleared by prom time next year."

6. Ms. Taylor has contracted genital herpes. Which of the following has the highest priority when teaching the client about the disease?
   A. Take the medication as ordered.
   B. Avoid oral sex.
   C. Wash hands before eating a meal.
   D. The disease is incurable.

7. A breast cancer client develops shingles following chemotherapy treatment. A priority nursing diagnosis for this client would be:
   A. Therapeutic Regimen Management, Ineffective.
   B. Disturbed Body Image.
   C. Deficient Knowledge.
   D. Self-Care Deficit.

8. Discharge instructions for a client diagnosed with cellulitis should include:
   A. apply cool compresses t.i.d.
   B. discontinue the medication when the symptoms disappear.
   C. cover draining lesions with a sterile dressing.
   D. keep skin moist at all times.

9. Mr. Yale is diagnosed with basal cell carcinoma of the left cheek. Which of the following indicates a need for further teaching?
   A. "I need to wear a hat when I go outside in the sun."
   B. "I need to get my affairs in order, since I don't have much time left."
   C. "The cancer can return after treatment."
   D. "The treatment is usually effective."

10. A neighbor calls during the evening and asks you to look at her child's head. When you asked about the problem, the neighbor says that "rice grains" are stuck to the roots of the hair. From your knowledge of lice, you would anticipate that a physician will diagnose:
    A. scabies.
    B. pediculosis corporis.
    C. pediculosis capitis.
    D. tinea pedis.

11. The nurse knows that another word used to describe dry skin is:
    A. pruritus.
    B. xerosis.
    C. xerostoma.
    D. cyanosis.

12. A common medication used in the treatment of acne is:
    A. Accutane.
    B. aspirin.
    C. Allopurinol.
    D. Arimidex.

13. Shingles is a viral infection also known as:
    A. herpes simplex 1.
    B. herpes simplex 2.
    C. herpes zoster.
    D. herpes simplex 4.

14. Which of the following is a parasite?
    A. Lice
    B. Warts
    C. Staphylococcus
    D. Streptococcus

15. A complementary therapy used to treat boils is:
    A. green root.
    B. licorice root.
    C. tea-tree oil.
    D. coffee bean oil.

Chapter 46

Caring for Clients With Burns

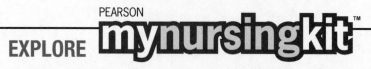

EXPLORE PEARSON mynursingkit™

MyNursingKit is your one stop for online chapter review materials and resources. Prepare for success with additional NCLEX®-style practice questions, interactive assignments and activities, web links, animations and videos, and more!

Register your access code from the front of your book at www.mynursingkit.com

KEY TERMS

Match each term with its appropriate definition.

_____ 1. Eschar
_____ 2. Superficial partial-thickness burn
_____ 3. Radiation burn
_____ 4. Full-thickness burn
_____ 5. Chemical burn
_____ 6. Electrical burn
_____ 7. Superficial
_____ 8. Deep partial-thickness burn
_____ 9. Debridement
_____ 10. Thermal burn

A. Results from acidic or basic agents
B. Entire dermis plus hair follicles
C. Removal of dead tissue from wound
D. Caused by brief exposure or contact
E. Exposure to dry heat
F. Hard crust that forms over wounds
G. Sunburn
H. Severity depends on duration of voltage
I. Extends to subcutaneous fat, muscle, bone
J. Involves only epidermis

LEARNING OUTCOMES

1. Define burns.

2. Describe the "rule of nines."

3. Describe Curling's ulcer.

4. Define debridement.

5. Identify initial focus assessments regarding major burns.

6. Identify nursing diagnoses regarding burn clients.

7. Define contracture.

8. Describe silver nitrate.

9. Identify diagnostic testing used to assess and monitor burns.

10. Define full-thickness burn.

APPLY WHAT YOU LEARNED

A 42-year-old male presents to the ER after being burned by a chemical at work. The burns only appear on the client's face. He was wearing goggles, hat, gloves, and long sleeves while working with this chemical.

1. Using the "rule of nines," what percentage of his body is burned?

2. What treatment would the nurse expect to see ordered?

MULTIPLE CHOICE

Circle the answer that best completes the following statements.

1. A client sustains second- and third-degree burns over 45% of his body. The nursing care immediately following this burn injury is:
   A. prevention of infection.
   B. fluid resuscitation.
   C. preservation of body image.
   D. maintenance of urinary output.

2. The nurse describes the client's burn injury in the medical record as "pale, waxy and moist, with large blister formation." The client states that the pain is at level 5. The depth of injury is most likely:
   A. full thickness.
   B. superficial.
   C. superficial partial thickness.
   D. deep partial thickness.

3. The emergent stage of burn injury treatment includes:
   A. closure of the burn wound.
   B. wound debridement.
   C. estimating the extent of the burn.
   D. skin grafting.

4. Mr. Andrews, age 68, is receiving fluid resuscitation of Ringer's lactate at 250 mL/hr. Which of the following indicates a complication of fluid therapy?
   A. Urinary output of 85 mL/hour
   B. Complaints of abdominal pain
   C. Crackles in lung bases
   D. Edema in the burn areas

5. A major complication of a severe burn is infection. If all of the following nursing interventions are placed on the care plan, which would be the highest priority?
   A. Monitor and record body temperature every two hours.
   B. Review WBC counts.
   C. Maintain a high-calorie diet.
   D. Use aseptic technique.

6. A 7-year-old child sustains a thermal burn to her face when she trips over an open gas heater. Your first action should be to:
   A. determine the depth of the burn.
   B. assess the respiratory status.
   C. provide pain medication.
   D. read the doctor's orders.

7. Your client is receiving Ensure at 60 mL/hr via a nasogastric tube. Which of the following interventions should be written on the nursing care plan?
   A. Record daily weights.
   B. Replace feeding tube every 24 hours.
   C. Administer a stool softener once a day.
   D. Increase the rate when the client complains of hunger.

8. Mrs. Jones has sustained burns over 55% of her body. She complains of nausea and has been throwing up a dark green fluid. Your next action would be to:
   A. assess bowel sounds.
   B. insert a nasogastric tube.
   C. administer an antiemetic.
   D. notify the charge nurse.

9. The nurse is reviewing the lab work for a client with severe burns over 60% of his body. The HGB is 10.8 and the HCT is 55%. The nurse recognizes that these lab values may indicate:
   A. blood loss.
   B. nutritional deficit.
   C. hemolysis and fluid shifts.
   D. infection.

10. A client is complaining of severe pain after receiving second- and third-degree burns to her chest and lower extremities. The nurse expects to administer medication by the:
   A. intravenous route.
   B. intramuscular route.
   C. subcutaneous route.
   D. oral route.

11. Silver nitrate wet dressings are used as a topical treatment for a client with a full-thickness burn to the left arm. Client teaching should include:
   A. the dressing will be painful.
   B. the dressing will be removed every two hours.
   C. the dressing will feel warm.
   D. the dressing will cause the skin to turn black.

12. The primary goal of the rehabilitative stage should be to:
   A. prevent contractures.
   B. prevent infection.
   C. manage the pain.
   D. increase the nutritional status.

13. You have been assigned to assist the physician in the debridement of a burn wound located on a client's forehead. Which of the following actions would not be appropriate for this client?
    A. Administer pain medications 30 minutes before the procedure.
    B. Wash the wound with Hibiclens.
    C. Provide a pair of surgical scissors to remove eschar.
    D. Trim any hair that might interfere with the procedure.

14. Mr. Kaiser will be going to surgery for a heterograft. He asks the nurse, "Where does the doctor get the graft material?" The nurse should state:
    A. "We have the local university tissue bank send a piece from a cadaver."
    B. "The surgeon will take a piece of skin from your thigh."
    C. "Your daughter has already volunteered to provide a graft."
    D. "The graft is usually taken from a pig skin."

15. A client with 60% burn injuries will be receiving a nutritional diet. You expect that the physician will initially order:
    A. a 2500 calorie, high-protein, high-carbohydrate, low-fat diet.
    B. TPN.
    C. enteral feedings through a small-bore tube.
    D. gastrostomy feedings.

Chapter 47

Mental Health and Assessment

KEY TERMS

Match each term with its appropriate definition.

_J_	1. Insight	A.	Chemical messengers that conduct impulses from one neuron to the next
_F_	2. Concrete thinking	B.	Attitudes, beliefs, customs, and behaviors passed from one generation to the next
_A_	3. Neurotransmitter	C.	Nerve cell
_C_	4. Neuron	D.	Self-understanding
_H_	5. Synapse	E.	Rapidly changing emotional expressions
_G_	6. Stigma	F.	Thought processes that are literal or without creativity
_I_	7. Psychosocial	G.	Negative attitude marking people with certain conditions as less valuable
_B_	8. Culture	H.	Space between the axon and its target cell's dendrite
_D_	9. Self-concept	I.	Refers to things that affect psychologic and social functioning
_E_	10. Labile	J.	How we relate to ourselves and to others

LEARNING OUTCOMES

1. Identify the seven aspects of a mentally healthy person.

2. Define insight.

3. Identify five neurotransmitters.

4. Describe a synapse.

5. Define stigma.

6. Describe psychological functions.

7. Identify the four self-concepts.

8. Identify the five most common mental illnesses.

9. Describe how mental illnesses are diagnosed.

10. Define concrete thinking.

APPLY WHAT YOU LEARNED

The student nurse is studying mental health. She understands that it is holistic and individualized. The assessment of a client with a suspected mental illness relies on subjective and objective data to evaluate the situation. A mental status assessment tool is also utilized for evaluation and treatment.

1. Identify parts included in a complete mental status assessment.

2. What nonjudgmental question could the nurse ask to find out why the client is presenting to the hospital?

MULTIPLE CHOICE

Circle the answer that best completes the following statements.

1. Nancy is a 22-year-old client diagnosed with depression. When assessing the client's past coping behaviors the nurse knows to ask:
    A. "Why are you depressed?"
    B. "When the stress gets really bad, what do you do?"
    C. "So, what happened this time?"
    D. "Don't you realize how blessed you are?"

2. A neurotransmitter thought to be decreased in depression is:
    A. GABA.
    B. norepinephrine.
    C. acetylcholine.
    D. FTGA.

3. To assess short-term memory, ask the client to remember three words when you begin the mental status assessment. If the client remembers accurately, short-term memory is said to be intact when you ask what the three words were:
    A. 10 seconds later.
    B. 30 minutes later.
    C. 5–10 minutes later.
    D. 5 hours later.

4. One way to assess abstract thinking ability is to ask the client to interpret a proverb. This simple assessment can shed light on the client's:
    A. thought process.
    B. emotional state.
    C. life experiences.
    D. behavior.

5. An inflated appraisal of one's abilities, power, or knowledge is termed:
    A. labile.
    B. neologism.
    C. euphoria.
    D. grandiosity.

6. A young woman comes into the clinic with chronic pancreatitis. She smiles when you tell a joke, but her overall affect is sad. Because nurses treat clients holistically, an important aspect of nursing in this case is to also promote:
   A. no pain.
   B. patient advocacy.
   C. physical strength.
   ✓ D. mental health.

7. Mental disorders are diagnosed according to the diagnostic criteria published in:
   A. *Taber's*.
   B. the *DHHS*.
   ✓ C. the *DSM-IV-TR*.
   D. the *PDR*.

8. The leading cause of disability in developed countries by 2020 is projected to be:
   A. psychosis.
   ✓ B. major depression.
   C. schizophrenia.
   D. anxiety.

9. In their role as client advocates, nurses should stop using negative labels about people who have mental illnesses, and:
   ✓ A. educate the public.
   B. have a staff meeting.
   C. preach to the choir.
   D. educate each other.

10. A more specific assessment that is appropriate for a client with mental disorders is called a:
    A. psychosocial assessment.
    B. complete assessment.
    ✓ C. mental status examination.
    D. focused examination.

11. To think without creativity is known as:
    ✓ A. concrete thinking.
    B. abstract thinking.
    C. foolish thinking.
    D. insight.

12. The nurse recognizes that which neurotransmitter is decreased in Alzheimer's disease?
    ✓ A. Serotonin
    B. GABA
    C. Acetylcholine
    D. Norepinephrine

13. All of the following are common mental illnesses except:
    A. schizophrenia.
    B. bipolar disorder.
    ✓ C. self-inflicted injuries.
    D. drug abuse.

14. What percentage of the population is affected by schizophrenia?
    A. 1.1%
    B. 5%
    C. 20%
    D. 40%

15. Diagnostic criteria are found in the:
    A. *PDR*.
    B. *DSMMD*.
    C. PMS.
    D. ESR.

Chapter 48

Caring for Clients With Cognitive Disorders

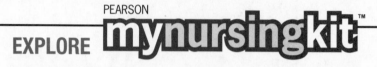

EXPLORE PEARSON mynursingkit™

MyNursingKit is your one stop for online chapter review materials and resources. Prepare for success with additional NCLEX®-style practice questions, interactive assignments and activities, web links, animations and videos, and more!

Register your access code from the front of your book at
www.mynursingkit.com

KEY TERMS

Match each term with its appropriate definition.

_____ 1. Cognition

_____ 2. Delirium

_____ 3. Aphasia

_____ 4. Dementia

_____ 5. Illusion

_____ 6. Sundowning

_____ 7. Procedural memory

_____ 8. Declarative memory

_____ 9. Reality orientation

_____ 10. Apraxia

A. Memory impairment and cognitive deficits that interfere with function

B. Temporary condition that alters the level of consciousness

C. Misinterpretation of environmental stimuli

D. Aspect of remembering that applies to skills or physical activities

E. Reminders of person, place, and time

F. Inability to perform complex movements

G. Aspect of remembering that involves facts and standard learning

H. Increased mental confusion in the evening

I. Partial or total inability to express and understand speech

J. Thinking skills

LEARNING OUTCOMES

1. Identify characteristics of normal memory lapse.

2. Describe manifestations regarding delirium.

3. Discuss components of the mini mental state exam.

4. Define agnosia.

5. Identify common causes of dementia.

6. Define Alzheimer's disease.

7. Identify risk factors for vascular dementia.

8. Discuss the differences between delirium and dementia.

9. Define hyperorality.

10. Identify medications used in dementia.

APPLY WHAT YOU LEARNED

While working in the neighborhood clinic, a nurse encounters a 68-year-old male who reports problems with misplacing keys and his watch. Upon further conversation, the nurse notices that the client can not recall the current day and is having problems selecting words for conversation.

1. What do the above signs and symptoms indicate?

2. What resources could be utilized for this client?

3. What nursing diagnoses would be appropriate for this client?

MULTIPLE CHOICE

Circle the answer that best completes the following statements.

1. The nurse knows that as the brain ages, it loses neurons, becomes smaller and:
   A. gains weight.
   B. loses weight.
   C. gains capacity.
   D. loses common sense.

2. All of the following are normal memory lapses except:
   A. momentarily forgetting the date.
   B. losing track of what you planned to say.
   C. forgetting where you left your keys.
   D. forgetting how to use numbers.

3. All of the following are frequent causes of delirium except:
   A. gout.
   B. heart disease.
   C. psychosocial stressors.
   D. infections.

4. What is the tool used to assess the mental state of clients?
   A. MSDS
   B. MDS
   C. MMSE
   D. MRSA

5. The nurse understands that the loss of comprehension of sensation is:
   A. aphasia.
   B. apraxia.
   C. agnosia.
   D. asystole.

6. The following are types of dementia except:
   A. vascular.
   B. Lewy body.
   C. Alzheimer's.
   D. congenital.

7. A client presents to the clinic with a history of smoking, HTN, hyperlipidemia, CAD, and DM. The nurse understands that this client is at risk for:
   A. vascular dementia.
   B. Lewy body dementia.
   C. Crohn's disease.
   D. Lou Gehrig's disease.

8. All are symptoms of delirium except:
   A. quick.
   B. slow.
   C. fluctuates.
   D. hyper-vigilant.

9. The nurse is speaking with a client who is having problems with language, memory loss, decreased judgment, and loss of initiative. These are symptoms of:
   A. Huntington's disease.
   B. Lewy body dementia.
   C. Lou Gehrig's disease.
   D. Alzheimer's disease.

10. Another term used for putting everything within reach into one's mouth is:
    A. hypersensitivity.
    B. hyperotitis.
    C. hyperacuity.
    D. hyperorality.

11. To confabulate is to:
    A. make aware.
    B. make a policy.
    C. make up stories.
    D. make contracts.

12. The nurse on the 3–11 shift notices that a 68-year-old female client has increased confusion after supper. The nurse understands this is characteristic of:
    A. wandering.
    B. sundowning.
    C. sunrising.
    D. depression.

13. The neurotransmitter that is decreased in Alzheimer's disease is:
    A. serotonin.
    B. acetylcholine.
    C. pepsin.
    D. leptin.

14. The nurse would expect a client with dementia to be taking the medication:
    A. Exelon.
    B. Excedrin.
    C. Effexor.
    D. Elavil.

15. The loss of brain tissue will have the following appearance on an MRI:
    A. localized folds.
    B. no folds.
    C. superficial folds.
    D. deep folds.

Chapter 49

Caring for Clients With Psychotic Disorders

KEY TERMS

Match each term with its appropriate definition.

_____ 1. Psychosis   A. Sensory perceptions that seem very real but occur without external stimuli

_____ 2. Schizophrenia   B. A complex disorder of the brain

_____ 3. Familial   C. A thought disorder that causes delusions, hallucinations, disorganized speech, or disorganized behavior

_____ 4. Hallucination   D. Early symptoms

_____ 5. Delusion   E. Fixed false beliefs

_____ 6. Alogia   F. Decreased amount and richness of speech

_____ 7. Avolition   G. Generalized muscle spasms that result in arching of the back and neck

_____ 8. Prodromal   H. Therapeutic environment

_____ 9. Milieu   I. A lack of motivation

_____ 10. Opisthotonos   J. Occurring in families

LEARNING OUTCOMES

1. Define psychosis.

2. Describe a hallucination.

3. Identify the four types of cognitive impairments.

4. Define affect.

5. Describe milieu therapy.

6. Identify nursing diagnoses related to psychotic disorders.

7. Identify some outcomes for a client with schizophrenia.

8. Define tardive dyskinesia.

9. Describe prodromal phases.

10. Describe bizarre delusions.

APPLY WHAT YOU LEARNED

An 18-year-old male presents to your clinic and tells you that he keeps seeing Santa Claus in his living room and everywhere he goes. The client states that he does not intend to harm himself or anyone else. He just wants Santa Claus to "go away."

1. What might be the diagnosis for this client?

2. How would the nurse interact with this client?

MULTIPLE CHOICE

Circle the answer that best completes the following statements.

1. The negative symptoms of schizophrenia involve a deficit or decrease of normal functions and include:
   A. volition.
   B. increased speech.
   C. anhedonia.
   D. sad affect.

2. Positive (or psychotic) symptoms seem to be an excess or distortion of normal functions and include:
   A. hallucinations and delusions.
   B. delusions and mania.
   C. mania and hallucinations.
   D. anxiety and delusions.

3. People with schizophrenia die earlier than other people do. The largest contributor to this excess mortality rate is:
   A. heart attack.
   B. suicide.
   C. cancer.
   D. renal failure.

4. The brain disorder in schizophrenia renders many affected people unable to understand that they are mentally ill. The percentage of people **NOT** receiving treatment at any given time because of lack of insight is:
   A. 90%.
   B. 40%.
   C. 54%.
   D. 11%.

5. A coexisting problem common in schizophrenia is:
   A. homelessness.
   B. anxiety.
   C. chronic disease.
   D. substance abuse.

6. For psychiatric inpatients, the therapeutic milieu should be:
   A. simple, safe, and restrictive.
   B. restrictive, flashing lights, and safe.
   C. tolerant, safe, and dependent.
   D. pleasant, simple, and safe.

7. Antipsychotic medications are used to treat disorders such as schizophrenia that are characterized by psychosis. These drugs are also called:
   A. neurostimulators.
   B. mood stabilizers.
   C. neuroleptics.
   D. anticonvulsants.

8. A young woman approaches you on the street asking for your forgiveness. She believes that you are a demon and screams loudly, "I know who you are! You talk to me all the time." You remember from your nursing class that schizophrenia may result in:
   A. craziness.
   B. delusions.
   C. denial.
   D. drinking.

9. Roger, age 28 and diagnosed with schizophrenia, stopped taking his medication. What percentage chance is there that he will relapse within a year?
   A. 80%
   B. 95%
   C. 0%
   D. 18%

10. It is important for clients on antipsychotic therapy to be assessed for abnormal involuntary movement with a scale such as:
    A. AIMS.
    B. MME.
    C. HESI.
    D. NCLEX.

11. The nurse recognizes that the client saying, "I am Spiderman" is:
    A. grandiose.
    B. delusion of reference.
    C. somatic.
    D. bizarre.

12. The phase in which the client experiences early symptoms before a full psychotic episode is:
    A. anhedonia.
    B. prodromal.
    C. preprandial.
    D. postprandial.

13. The nurse understands that signs of EPS include all but:
    A. dystonia.
    B. dyskinesia.
    C. akathisia.
    D. dysuria.

14. In understanding the effects of antipsychotics, the nurse knows that:
    A. it may take up to 4 weeks or longer.
    B. it may take up to 2 days.
    C. it may take up to 6 months.
    D. it may take up to 1 year.

15. The inability to sit still is known as:
    A. akathisia.
    B. dysphagia.
    C. arthralgia.
    D. dystonia.

Chapter 50

Caring for Clients With Mood Disorders

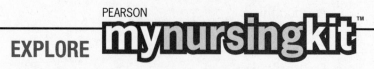

EXPLORE **mynursingkit**™

MyNursingKit is your one stop for online chapter review materials and resources. Prepare for success with additional NCLEX®-style practice questions, interactive assignments and activities, web links, animations and videos, and more!

Register your access code from the front of your book at **www.mynursingkit.com**

KEY TERMS

Match each term with its appropriate definition.

D 1. Mood
A. Normal range of emotions

C 2. Affect
B. Inability to feel pleasure

A 3. Euthymic
C. The emotions a person is currently expressing

G 4. Hypersomnia
D. A pervasive and sustained emotion that influences how a person perceives the world

H 5. Phototherapy
E. A mental disorder

B 6. Anhedonia
F. Abnormal or excessive dilation of the pupils

E 7. Depression
G. Sleeping too much

F 8. Mydriasis
H. Light therapy

J 9. Manic speech
I. Period of persistently elevated, expansive, or irritable mood

I 10. Mania
J. Rapid and pressured

LEARNING OUTCOMES

1. Define mood.

2. Identify risk factors for depression.

3. Describe psychomotor agitation.

4. Identify protective factors for suicide.

5. Define suicide.

6. Identify side effects related to anticholinergic drugs.

7. Identify foods to avoid when taking MAOIs.

8. Define ECT.

9. Describe manifestations regarding bipolar disorder.

10. Identify side effects of lithium.

APPLY WHAT YOU LEARNED

A 62-year-old female has been widowed for about one year and suffered a recent stroke which left her paralyzed on her left side. She is currently residing in a nursing home and has no other family. She does not leave her room and keeps telling staff members that she wishes "God would take me already."

1. How would the nurse talk to this client who is feeling hopeless?

2. What is the first question the nurse should ask this client?
   Are you thinking of quiting yourself.

MULTIPLE CHOICE

Circle the answer that best completes the following statements.

1. Diane, 30, comes into the clinic stating, "I'm so depressed!" The nurse knows that the diagnostic criteria for a major depressive episode include that the client must have at least five symptoms during:
   A. 10 days.
   ✓B. a 2-week period.
   C. a 3-month period.
   D. 20 days.

2. A recent advance in brain imaging that shows abnormal function in the prefrontal cortex of the cerebrum and in the limbic system during depressive episodes is called:
   ✓A. PET.
   B. CAT.
   C. EEG.
   D. PCT.

3. A major life stressor precedes the first major depressive episode for many people. The average age of onset is in the:
   A. teenage years.
   B. mid-30s.
   ✓C. mid-20s.
   D. senior years.

4. Only 12% of people are willing to take medication for depression, while _____ would take medication for a headache:
   A. 50%
   B. 92%
   C. 36%
   ✓D. 70%

5. The nurse knows that it is important to educate clients, their families, and communities about depression, its outcomes, and treatments. Knowledge can help people comply with treatment, be free from unnecessary guilt, and maintain:
   A. a healthy lifestyle.
   B. their jobs.
   C. faith.
   ✓D. hope.

6. More Americans die each year from suicide than from homicide. An average of 85 Americans die from suicide each day. Suicide rates are highest among:
   A. older adults.
   B. children.
   C. teenagers.
   D. middle-aged adults.

7. Most antidepressants act on two major brain neurotransmitters which regulate mood:
   A. serotonin and dopamine
   B. GABA and norepinephrine
   C. serotonin and norepinephrine
   D. norepinephrine and dopamine

8. Clients tend to have better outcomes when they are treated with a combination of medications and:
   A. group therapy.
   B. psychotherapy.
   C. music therapy.
   D. cognitive therapy.

9. Unwarranted optimism, grandiosity, and poor judgment characterize:
   A. Depressive Disorder.
   B. Paranoid Disorder.
   C. Sleep Disorder.
   D. Bipolar Disorder.

10. Psychosocial factors are important in the timing of manic episodes, and stressful events may precede them. Mania is a:
    A. physical condition.
    B. medicinal condition.
    C. biologic condition.
    D. mental condition.

11. The nurse understands that if a client is euthymic, the client is:
    A. in the normal range.
    B. psychotic.
    C. depressed.
    D. irritated.

12. A client who is experiencing no pleasure is suffering from:
    A. psychomotor retardation.
    B. anhedonia.
    C. psychomotor agitation.
    D. depression.

13. An average of how many Americans die from suicide each day?
    A. 50
    B. 100
    C. 85
    D. 245

14. The nurse understands that treatments with ECT induce:
    A. generalized seizures.
    B. generalized depression.
    C. generalized paralysis.
    D. generalized weakness.

15. The term pressured speech is used to describe:
    A. stress.
    B. depression.
    C. anger.
    D. mania.

Chapter 51

Caring for Clients With Anxiety Disorders

KEY TERMS

Match each term with its appropriate definition.

C	1. Anxiety	A.	A recurrent and intrusive thought that causes marked distress
I	2. Dysphoric	B.	An episode of intense fear or discomfort
B	3. Panic attack	C.	A feeling of uneasiness and activation of the autonomic nervous system in response to a vague, nonspecific threat
J	4. Paresthesia	D.	The quality of being hardy or "stress resistant"
E	5. Agoraphobia	E.	Anxiety about being in places or situations where escape may be difficult
A	6. Obsession	F.	A persistent and irrational fear
H	7. Compulsion	G.	Conscious ways that people deal with stress
F	8. Phobia	H.	Repetitive behavior that a person feels driven to perform
G	9. Coping	I.	Uncomfortable and distressed
D	10. Resilience	J.	Numbness or tingling

LEARNING OUTCOMES

1. Define anxiety.

2. Identify factors present with a panic attack.

3. Define posttraumatic stress disorder.

4. Identify medical conditions associated with anxiety.

5. Define paradoxical.

6. Describe resilience.

7. Identify antianxiety agents.

8. Define phobia.

9. Describe OCD.

10. Define coping behaviors.

APPLY WHAT YOU LEARNED

A 32-year-old male presents to the clinic shortly after being honorably discharged from the Air Force. He has a flat affect and tells you that his mind is "all over the place." He has trouble sleeping and states he is having nightmares.

1. What does the nurse suspect is the diagnosis?

2. What are some treatments appropriate for this client?

MULTIPLE CHOICE

Circle the answer that best completes the following statements.

1. A nursing assistant catheterized the wrong client. The nurse takes her aside to point out her error. This is an example of:
    A. adaptive behavior.
    B. favoritism.
    C. maladaptive behavior.
    D. prejudice.

2. George comes to the clinic convinced he is having a heart attack. He says the symptoms started on the way to a very important job interview. You suspect George is:
    A. having a case of nerves.
    B. looking for attention.
    C. having a panic attack.
    D. procrastinating.

3. A client copes with anxiety by deliberately relaxing or practicing deep breathing in situations that are expected to provoke anxiety, thereby interrupting the automatic anxiety responses. This client is using:
    A. ACT.
    B. ADHD.
    C. CBT.
    D. CHF.

4. CBT or behavioral therapy usually takes about:
    A. 1 month.
    B. 3 years.
    C. 2 weeks.
    D. 12 weeks.

5. Mr. Tracy demonstrates frequent mood changes. These changes are termed:
    A. anxiety.
    B. labile.
    C. euphoria.
    D. depression.

6. Martha comes into the doctor's office visibly upset. You talk to her and notice that she is unaware of her anxiety. All of her VS are increased and she has pressured speech. Martha is exhibiting what level of anxiety?
   A. Mild
   B. Severe
   ✓C. Panic
   D. Moderate

7. The limbic structure responsible for coordinating actions of the autonomic nervous system and endocrine system, and which is involved in control of emotions, nurturing behavior, and fear conditioning, is called the:
   A. hypothalamus.
   B. thalamus.
   ✓C. amygdala.
   D. pituitary.

8. Your client has learned to verbalize his own feelings of anxiety and understand his stress response. This phase of anxiety is called:
   A. family.
   B. community.
   ✓ C. stabilization.
   D. acute.

9. Nurses can diagnose and treat the symptom of anxiety:
   A. with M.D. orders only.
   B. with health care team approval.
   C. collaboratively.
   ✓D. independently.

10. Information about the client's usual coping methods can be helpful in:
    A. administering medicine.
    B. gaining information.
    C. discharge planning.
    ✓D. planning care.

11. The nurse understands that the hippocampus is responsible for:
    ✓ A. processing information between parts of the brain.
    B. composing neurons that produce hormones.
    C. coordinating action of ANS.
    D. relaying sensory input from spinal cord.

12. A client who has a widened perceptual field and increased ability to see relationships among data is in which state of anxiety?
    A. Panic
    B. Severe
    C. Moderate
    ✓D. Mild

13. When someone fears being out in a crowd, they suffer from:
    ✓A. agoraphobia.
    B. apiphobia.
    C. astraphobia.
    D. aviophobia.

14. Intrusive thoughts that cause distress are:
    A. compulsions
    B. obsessions ✓
    C. psychoses
    D. phobias

15. Which of the following is a sedative-hypnotic agent?
    A. Valium
    B. Xanax
    C. Restoril ✓
    D. Tranxene

Chapter 52

Caring for Clients With Personality Disorders

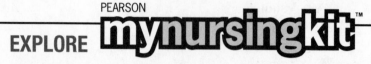

EXPLORE **mynursingkit**™

PEARSON

MyNursingKit is your one stop for online chapter review materials and resources. Prepare for success with additional NCLEX®-style practice questions, interactive assignments and activities, web links, animations and videos, and more!

Register your access code from the front of your book at
www.mynursingkit.com

KEY TERMS

Match each term with its appropriate definition.

_____ 1. Personality

_____ 2. Self-identity

_____ 3. Impulsive

_____ 4. Inflexibility

_____ 5. Stern

_____ 6. Linehan

_____ 7. Self-invalidation

_____ 8. Active passivity

_____ 9. Depersonalization

_____ 10. Parasuicidal

A. Behavior aimed at harming oneself

B. First used the term "borderline personality" in 1938

C. The psychosocial traits and characteristics that make a person an individual

D. A part of normal personality development

E. Leading contemporary theorist on Borderline Personality Disorder

F. An alteration in the perception of the self in which the client feels like she is looking at herself from outside her body

G. Unable to foresee consequences or control urges

H. Inability to change behavior when circumstances suggest that a change is indicated

I. Failure to recognize own emotions, thoughts, behaviors

J. Failure to work actively on solving own life problems

LEARNING OUTCOMES

1. Define personality.

2. Describe the three clusters.

3. Define inappropriate affect.

4. Define antisocial personality disorder.

5. Describe narcissistic personality disorder.

6. Describe dependent personality disorder.

7. Identify coping mechanisms for someone who suffers from self-harm.

8. Define borderline personality.

9. Define parasuicidal behavior.

10. Describe ideas of reference.

APPLY WHAT YOU LEARNED

The student nurse is studying personality disorders. The student will be observing clients with personality disorders in clinical next week. The objective for this rotation is to ensure safety within the unit for the clients and staff.

1. How will the student nurse prevent personality disordered clients from upsetting the unit?

MULTIPLE CHOICE

Circle the answer that best completes the following statements.

1. When teaching client strategies about coping with stress, the nurse uses the mnemonic: Wise mind ACCEPTS. The S stands for:
    A. stimulants are great.
    B. supine position works.
    C. sensations that are intense.
    D. Serax works wonders.

2. Which technique is used to help people who have used self-harm for coping find more enduring and adaptive ways to comfort themselves?
    A. Caffeine
    B. Five senses exercise
    C. Finger paints
    D. Valium

3. A nursing intervention for clients who have thoughts about self-harm or suicide is:
    A. negotiating a no-self-harm contract.
    B. administering sedatives.
    C. allowing two visitors every 30 minutes.
    D. maintaining a dimly lit, quiet room.

4. A pervasive pattern of social shyness, feelings of inadequacy, and hypersensitivity to negative evaluation is called:
    A. Avoidant Personality Disorder.
    B. anxiety.
    C. paranoid behavior.
    D. Schizotypal Personality Disorder.

5. Mrs. Jones demonstrates a need to be taken care of. This characterizes:
    A. Dependent Personality Disorder.
    B. anxiety.
    C. Affective Disorder.
    D. depression.

6. Marsha, 38, seems overly trusting of her boss. She believes everything her boss tells her and acts on any suggestions she makes. She has alienated all her friends because of her attempts to get attention by whatever means possible. The nurse suspects that Marsha suffers from:
    A. Narcissistic Personality Disorder.
    B. Dependent Personality Disorder.
    C. an addiction.
    D. Histrionic Personality Disorder.

7. Nurses can help people with personality disorders achieve:
    A. emotional well-being.
    B. great things.
    C. personal growth.
    D. a steady income.

8. Any judgment about a client's personality must take into account that person's ethnic, social, and:
   A. monetary background.
   B. cultural background.
   C. emotional background.
   D. psychologic background.

9. A client comes to the clinic crying, "I just left my boyfriend . . . he beat me every day, I just couldn't take it any more. I'm so weak; maybe if I could take it he would love me more." As a nurse you know the best response would be:
   A. "Are you crazy?"
   B. "If you go back, he will continue to harm you."
   C. "He is an adult and responsible for his own behavior."
   D. "Why do you want to go back?"

10. One way a nurse can prevent a client with personality disorder from disrupting the unit is by:
    A. making the unit rules clear.
    B. having a conference with staff.
    C. A and B.
    D. none of the above.

11. The nurse knows that a client who suffers from OCD is in which cluster?
    A. Fearful
    B. Eccentric
    C. Dramatic
    D. Odd

12. Someone who laughs when a person dies suffers from:
    A. delusions.
    B. inappropriate affect.
    C. psychomotor agitation.
    D. depression.

13. Avoidant personality disorder is characterized by:
    A. social isolation.
    B. anxiety.
    C. powerlessness.
    D. fear.

14. The relatively stable way in which a person thinks, feels, and behaves is:
    A. personality.
    B. egocentric.
    C. selfish.
    D. normal.

15. When talking with a client who has a disturbed thought process, always:
    A. speak loudly and clearly.
    B. laugh and joke.
    C. reassure them of their safety.
    D. reassure them of their discharge.

Chapter 53

Caring for Clients With Substance Abuse or Dependency

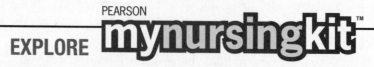

EXPLORE PEARSON **mynursingkit**™

MyNursingKit is your one stop for online chapter review materials and resources. Prepare for success with additional NCLEX®-style practice questions, interactive assignments and activities, web links, animations and videos, and more!

Register your access code from the front of your book at **www.mynursingkit.com**

KEY TERMS

Match each term with its appropriate definition.

_____ 1. Tolerance

_____ 2. Addiction

_____ 3. Denial

_____ 4. Intoxication

_____ 5. Wernicke's

_____ 6. Ataxia

_____ 7. Withdrawal

_____ 8. Blackout

_____ 9. Korsakoff's

_____ 10. Euphoria

A. Staggering gait

B. Exaggerated feeling of well-being

C. Experienced when use of a substance is discontinued

D. Symptoms caused by vitamin B deficiency

E. Inability to remember events that occurred during intoxicated state

F. Refusal to acknowledge existence of a situation or feeling

G. Increasing amounts of substance needed to create an effect

H. Mental and physical drug-seeking behaviors

I. Group of reversible symptoms produced by a substance

J. Alcoholic encephalopathy

LEARNING OUTCOMES

1. Define denial.

2. Identify commonly abused substances.

3. Identify withdrawal symptoms for alcoholism.

4. Define Korsakoff's syndrome.

5. Define Wernicke's syndrome.

6. Identify manifestations of fetal alcohol syndrome.

7. Define detoxification.

8. Describe rehabilitation.

9. Describe dual diagnosis.

10. Describe an impaired nurse.

APPLY WHAT YOU LEARNED

The student nurse is preparing for her community service project. She is required to attend an AA meeting and observe the steps involved. She is feeling a little nervous and does not know what to expect.

1. What stereotypes are created regarding alcoholics?

2. How would the student nurse assess for substance abuse?

MULTIPLE CHOICE

Circle the answer that best completes the following statements.

1. Drugs that distort the user's perception of reality are called:
   A. stimulants.
   B. amphetamines.
   C. hallucinogens.
   D. nicotine.

2. A medication given during alcohol withdrawal to prevent Wernicke–Korsakoff's syndrome is:
   A. caffeine.
   B. vitamin B_1.
   C. Dilantin.
   D. Valium.

3. A nursing intervention that provides low stimulation for the client during drug withdrawal includes:
   A. restricting visitors.
   B. administering sedatives.
   C. allowing two visitors every 30 minutes.
   D. maintaining a dimly lit, quiet room.

4. A drug prescribed to deter clients from drinking alcohol is:
   A. Antabuse.
   B. methadone.
   C. ReVia.
   D. Catapres.

5. Mr. Jones demonstrates frequent mood changes with increased alcohol intake. These changes are termed:
   A. labile.
   B. anxiety.
   C. euphoria.
   D. depression.

6. A young male increases his consumption of alcohol from one six-pack to two six-packs of beer per day to achieve the same effects. This action may indicate:
    A. addiction.
    B. intoxication.
    C. tolerance.
    D. dependence.

7. A local maintenance man is frequently seen drinking for hours at the local bar. He refuses to socialize with his neighbors and has been labeled an "angry man." The nurse is aware that the crucial phase of alcohol addiction includes:
    A. emotional and physical disintegration.
    B. memory blackouts.
    C. loss of control over the decision to drink or not to drink.
    D. a steady increase of alcohol consumption.

8. You remember from your nursing class that the chronic phase of alcohol addiction may result in:
    A. job loss.
    B. suicide.
    C. denial.
    D. drinking in secret.

9. A chronic alcoholic has been admitted to the medical floor for a laceration of the forehead and observation. During your physical assessment you note the presence of ascites, yellow skin, and severe muscle weakness. You suspect that this client may be diagnosed with end-stage liver disease known as:
    A. hepatic encephalopathy.
    B. alcoholic hepatitis.
    C. cirrhosis.
    D. portal hypertension.

10. A 21-year-old male was brought to the emergency room by the paramedics. They report the client was found, unresponsive, lying on a park bench. Their initial assessment noted pinpoint pupils and depressed respirations. The ER nurse suspects that this client may have overdosed on:
    A. alcohol.
    B. amphetamines.
    C. cocaine.
    D. heroin.

11. A client is concerned about the withdrawal effects from his use of the drug Ecstasy. He states, "I don't want to start shaking. I've seen it happen with my friend who drank too much." The best response by the nurse would be:
    A. "Don't worry, we'll be right here to watch you."
    B. "You won't have any withdrawal symptoms."
    C. "You should have stopped taking the drug a long time ago."
    D. "You won't have withdrawal symptoms, but you might have flashbacks."

12. At a chemical substance treatment center, the nurse is teaching the family about the importance of understanding drug withdrawal from heroin. He explains that a synthetic opiate will be used to replace the heroin. This drug is known as:
    A. methadone.
    B. naltrexone.
    C. Antabuse.
    D. Catapres.

13. You observe that the medication nurse always seems to go the bathroom after administering narcotics. You also notice that more pain medications are given when that particular nurse is on duty. Your next action should be to:
    A. do nothing; it is none of your business.
    B. confront the nurse when she comes out of the bathroom.
    C. discuss your concerns with your supervisor.
    D. continue to watch for more unusual behaviors.

14. The major goal of withdrawal management is:
    A. cessation of drug use.
    B. protection of society.
    C. physiological safety.
    D. maintaining sobriety.

15. The nurse establishes a nursing diagnosis of Deficient Knowledge for a client during the acute phase of substance abuse treatment. Teaching should include all of the following except:
    A. consequences of drug use.
    B. reasons behind drug use.
    C. coping strategies.
    D. recommended amounts of drug use.

Answer Key

Chapter 1 Nursing in the 21st Century

Matching

1. H ✓
2. C ✓
3. J ✓
4. A ✓
5. B ✓

6. D ✓
7. I ✓
8. E ✓
9. F ✓
10. G ✓

Learning Outcomes

1. Care of adults to promote and maintain health, and, during illness, to alleviate suffering. The focus is on the adult client's response to actual or potential disruptions in health.
2. Eliminating preventable disease, achieving health equity, and promoting healthy development and health behaviors across every stage of life are some leading health indicators for Healthy People 2020.
3. The process of evaluating, monitoring, or regulating the standard of services provided to the consumer.
4. Objectives of an advocate are to communicate with other healthcare team members, provide teaching to client and family, support clinical decision making, suggest referrals as appropriate, and identify community resources.
5. Phases of the nursing process are: Assessment, Nursing Diagnosis, Planning, Implementation, and Evaluation.
6. Critical thinking is a process used by nurses to determine a client's needs and is based on priority. The nurse uses knowledge and experience to develop the appropriate interventions in order to assist the client to maintain an optimum state of wellness.
7. Components of the LPN/LVN Scope of Practice include: collecting data, participating in the plan of care, maintaining safe and effective nursing care, promoting a safe and therapeutic environment, communicating with other healthcare professionals, and continuing education.
8. The purpose of HIPAA is to protect each individual's health information while allowing such information to be shared as needed for effective care. By protecting this information, the client's privacy and dignity are maintained.
9. Ethics is a set of principles of conduct that are concerned with moral duty, values, obligations, and the distinction between right and wrong.

10. Professional boundaries are the limits maintained between a person who is vulnerable and the person who has the power. It is the nurse's responsibility to establish and maintain professional boundaries while retaining an appropriate level of involvement for effective care.

Apply What You Learned

1. The phases of the nursing process are: Assessment, where data is collected; Nursing Diagnosis, where a conclusion is developed concerning condition; Planning, where interventions and outcomes are designed; Implementation, carrying out the plan; and Evaluation, where goals are analyzed to see if revision or completion has been met.
2. During the evaluation phase, the nurse determines whether or not the plan was effective. Then it is decided if the same plan is to continue, be revised, or terminated. It is based upon the expected outcomes that were established during the planning phase. Evaluation takes place continuously throughout care.
3. First of all, only a physician can develop a medical diagnosis. A nurse develops a nursing diagnosis in order to assist the client is achieving optimum wellness given the current condition. A medical diagnosis will tell the nurse what the disease is, while a nursing diagnosis will guide the planning of a client's health care status.

Multiple Choice

1. C
2. D
3. A
4. D
5. B

6. A
7. D
8. A
9. C
10. A

11. C
12. A
13. D
14. A
15. B

Chapter 2 Health, Illness, and Settings of Care

Matching

1. J
2. A
3. E
4. B
5. I

6. C
7. H
8. D
9. F
10. G

Learning Outcomes

1. The health–illness continuum is a representation of health as a dynamic process, with high-level wellness at one extreme of the continuum and death at the opposite extreme. Individuals place themselves at different locations on the continuum at specific points in time.

2. Homeostasis is the body's tendency to maintain a dynamic steady state or balance under constantly changing conditions.

3. Illness is the response a person has to a disease. This response is highly individualized because the person responds not only to his or her own perceptions of the disease, but also to the perceptions of others.

4. Some characteristics of a chronic illness include: It is permanent, it leaves a permanent disability, it is caused by nonreversible pathologic alterations, it requires special teaching of the client for rehabilitation and it may require a long period of care.

5. Long-term care is for people who are mentally or physically unable to care for themselves independently and may require health care and help with activities of daily living. Clients may remain in these types of facilities for the rest of their lives.

6. Community-based nursing is care that focuses on culturally competent individuals who can help families with their healthcare needs. It can occur in clinics, day care programs, churches, schools, and correctional facilities.

7. Community-based nursing care settings include: county health departments, parish nursing, homeless shelters, crisis intervention centers, ambulatory surgical centers, free clinics, hospice care, and prisons.

8. Clients who would benefit from home healthcare services are those who cannot live alone because of age, illness, or disability. They may also have a chronic disease or be terminally ill and want to die in their home with comfort and dignity. They do not require inpatient treatment but need assistance such as an outpatient surgical client might require.

9. Areas to assess for safety in the home include: stairs, smoke, bathroom safety equipment, throw rugs, expired medications, inappropriate footwear, inadequate food supply, and poorly functioning utilities.

10. Suggestions for effective home care include: establishing trust, assessing the overall environment, promoting the client's ability to learn, paying attention to the client's needs, and being flexible.

Apply What You Learned

1. The nurse needs to teach the client about bathroom safety equipment and perhaps have a bedside commode to be utilized on the first floor of the home. The nurse also needs to assess the lighting in the house and open the blinds for better visualization. Ask the client to repeat instructions to the nurse to verify understanding.

2. The nurse could recommend a senior center so that the client can make friends and have companionship, and a Meals-on-Wheels program to ensure that the client is being fed, as well as home health nursing visits.

Multiple Choice

1.	A ✓	6.	D ✓	11.	C ✓
2.	D ✓	7.	A ✓	12.	D ✓
3.	D ✓	8.	B ✓	13.	D
4.	C ✓	9.	B ✓	14.	C ✓
5.	C ✓	10.	D ✓	15.	B ✓

Chapter 3 Cultural and Developmental Considerations for Adults

Matching

1. C ✓
2. J ✓
3. A ✓
4. B ✓
5. I ✓

6. D ✓
7. E ✓
8. H ✓
9. G ✓
10. F ✓

Learning Outcomes

1. Culture includes: learned behavior, values, beliefs, norms, and practices that are shared by a particular group of people.
2. Health disparities are differences in the incidence and outcomes of diseases and disorders that occur among specific population groups in the United States.
3. Blood transfusions are not allowed, but will accept autologous blood transfusions. Avoid foods to which blood has been added, such as lunch-meats. Jehovah's Witnesses do not observe national or religious holidays.
4. Health risks for young adults include: motor vehicle crashes, use of firearms, substance abuse, sexually transmitted infections, drowning, fire, and occupational accidents.
5. Family carries out the tasks that are necessary for its survival and continuity such as: providing shelter, food, clothing, and healthcare; sharing money, time, and space; determining the roles and responsibilities of each member and ensuring socialization of members.
6. Ethnocentrism is a person's belief that their own cultural group's beliefs and values are the only acceptable ones.
7. Components of communication include: language, non-verbal cues, listening attentively, touching, and facial expression.
8. Personal space is importance because it allows the client to establish trust with the healthcare provider. It provides security, privacy, and a sense of control. Maintaining a comfort zone is important for the client to be able to communicate more freely, and thus improves care outcomes.
9. Social orientation includes a group of beliefs, values, and attitudes about important life events such as birth, death, puberty, childbearing, raising children, illness, and disease.
10. Health risks for middle adults include: maintaining a healthy weight, cardiovascular disease, cancer, substance abuse, and psychosocial stressors.

Apply What You Learned

1. Extended families, skip-generation families, alternative families, and blended families are all represented.
2. These students could be taught the importance of a healthy diet in order to prevent obesity, cardiovascular disease, and even certain cancers. They should also be taught about the appropriate amount of sleep to maintain health. Socialization should be taught in order for successful development into adulthood. This age group should also be taught about accident prevention, which will include sports and recreation, and STI prevention.

Multiple Choice

1.	D	6.	C	11.	A
2.	D	7.	B	12.	D
3.	A	8.	C	13.	B
4.	B	9.	B	14.	A
5.	A	10.	C	15.	C

Chapter 4 The Older Adult in Health and Illness

Matching

1.	J	6.	B
2.	C	7.	D
3.	E	8.	H
4.	A	9.	I
5.	G	10.	F

Learning Outcomes

1. Ageism is a form of prejudice in which older adults are stereotyped by characteristics found only in a small number of their age group. Two myths related to older adults are that most older adults live in nursing homes, when in fact only about 5% do, and that most older adults are sick when in fact almost half of all older adults rate their health as good or excellent.

2. Gerontologic nursing is a specialty area in the care of the older adult. Research indicates that the older adult population is increasing more rapidly than any other age group, therefore increasing the demand for this specialty.

3. Cognition is the ability to perceive and understand one's world. It does not normally change with aging. Older adults may take longer to process information and to respond, they rely on lists and calendars more, and processing information is delayed when in a new environment.

4. Erikson would identify the older adult to be in the ego integrity vs. despair and disgust stage. This is where the older adult reflects on their life and accepts the past.

5. To encourage reminiscence, the nurse would begin by asking open-ended questions to get the older adult to speak about life events. The nurse could also ask the older adult to look at pictures and tell a story related to that picture.

6. Age-related physical changes in the older adult can include the hair on the scalp thinning, decreased turgor and dryness of the skin, narrowed visual field decreased sense of smell, decreased cardiac output, decreased gag reflex, and the liver decreases in weight and storage capacity.

7. Psychosocial changes are life changes affecting relationships, income, or location. Widowhood and retirement are two of the most significant life changes, which the older adult must deal with and accept.

8. In teaching the older adult about prevention of accidents, remind them to install smoke detectors, not to use throw rugs, have adequate lighting, and to always wear corrective lenses and hearing aids when driving.

9. Alzheimer's disease is the most common degenerative neurologic illness. Symptoms usually seen in the early stages are loss of concentration and forgetfulness. It is not considered a normal part of aging.

10. To improve or maintain an older adult's quality of life, it is important for them to eat a healthy diet, not use tobacco products, receive immunizations for the flu, and continue with annual screenings to detect chronic illnesses.

Apply What You Learned

1. Instruct the client and family to keep the house well lit and free of throw rugs. Install smoke detectors and use hand railings in the bathroom/tub areas.

2. When promoting the health of the older adult, it is important to assess mobility for exercising, verify if they have dentures or loose/damaged teeth, review their diet for fiber and fluid intake, discuss neighborhood safety and community events, and evaluate that they have a clean, odor-free environment.

3. Since the client lives alone, the nurse should ask the social services department to speak with her to make sure that the home is ready and safe for her return. The nurse should also have the dietician speak with her regarding a low sodium diet related to the hypertension. Another possibility would be for someone from the physical therapy department to give her exercise tips to assist in the reduction of blood pressure.

Multiple Choice

1.	C	6.	A	11.	C
2.	A	7.	A	12.	C
3.	B	8.	D	13.	D
4.	B	9.	C	14.	B
5.	C	10.	B	15.	A

Chapter 5 Guidelines for Client Assessment

Key Terms

1.	D	6.	A
2.	I	7.	C
3.	B	8.	G
4.	F	9.	H
5.	E	10.	J

Learning Outcomes

1. The purpose of a client assessment is to collect subjective and objective data, to collect information about the client's family and community, to identify past and present behaviors regarding health care, and to identify data that may suggest risk or actual health problems.

2. Subjective data, or symptoms, are experiences only the client can describe, such as nausea and pain. Objective data, or signs, are observable and measurable pieces of information, such as vital signs and lab results.

3. Components in a health history would include: biographical data, reason for health care visit, history of present illness, past medical and surgical history, family history, and lifestyle.

4. There are four methods to physical examination: inspection, palpation, percussion, and auscultation.

5. Some assessment findings in the older adult would include: dry skin, loss of hair pigment, cataracts, decreased hearing, loss of teeth, increased blood pressure, decreased bowel sounds, decreased range of motion, stooped posture, and slower response to questions.

6. When assessing the pupils, use a penlight to observe the reaction to light, check for constriction or accommodation, and verify the presence of convergence.

7. Bradycardia exists when the heart rate is slow, usually below 60 beats per minute. Tachycardia is when the heart rate is fast, usually above 100 beats per minute.

8. The amplitude of the pulse refers to the strength of the pulse. It can be 0 which means absent, 1+ which indicates thready and not easily palpated, 2+ is weak, 3+ is normal and palpated easily and 4+ is bounding with strong pulsations.

9. To evaluate mental status, ask the client about a person, place, time, and situation. Also verify if they are alert and awake, lethargic, stuporous, or perhaps comatose.

10. To document accurately, write information down as soon as possible, be legible, organize the data, avoid judgments, record findings, use approved abbreviations, and be sure to be logical in the way the documentation flows.

Apply What You Learned

1. Objective data can be seen, heard, touched, or smelled. Appearance of client's clothes and overall hygiene can be considered objective.

2. Subjective data are experiences only the client can describe. "Little joy in activities" and "loss of appetite" are subjective.

3. Initially, the nurse should focus the assessment on safety. Does the client have plans to cause harm to himself or others? If not, maintain the focus on the client's mental status. Due to the data presented, the client may need a consultation with a mental health professional.

Multiple Choice

1. A ✓	6. D ✓	11. A ✓
2. B ✓	7. A ✓	12. D ✓
3. C	8. B	13. A
4. D	9. A	14. A ✓
5. D	10. B ✓	15. B

Chapter 6 Essential Nursing Pharmacology

Key Terms

1. B ✓
2. J ✓
3. H ✓
4. A ✓
5. D ✓
6. F ✓
7. C ✓
8. G ✓
9. E ✓
10. I ✓

Learning Outcomes

1. The six rights of medication administration are: right drug, client/patient, dose, route, time, and documentation.
2. Absorption is the first step in the passage of a drug through the body. It occurs from the time it enters the body until it reaches the bodily fluids that carry the drug to the site of action. Excretion is when the drugs are eliminated in the urine. The kidney is the most important organ of drug excretion.
3. The four names given to drugs are chemical, which includes the molecular structure of the drug; generic, which is the shorter version of the chemical name; trade, which is sometimes called the brand name and is usually trademarked or registered; and the official name, which is usually the trade name.
4. The purpose of a loading dose is to administer a higher-than-normal dose initially to quickly produce the desired result.
5. Idiosyncratic is when a very small percent of the population develops an unusual or unexpected response. Toxic is harmful, undesired effects or possibility of organ damage.
6. Agonists are drugs that combine with specific receptors to cause pharmacologic responses. Antagonists are drugs that prevent a receptor response or block normal cellular responses.
7. Polypharmacy is the use of many prescribed and over-the-counter drugs at the same time. This practice has been proven to be responsible for 15–20% of hospitalizations related to adverse medication reactions in older adults.
8. Age, body weight, genetics, ethnicity, disease conditions, and emotional state are some variables that affect drug responses.
9. Synergism is when two drugs are given together to cause a greater response than each one given separately, while potentiation is when the action of one drug increases the effect of the second drug.
10. Medication history components would include the use of over-the-counter and herbal drugs, alcohol consumption, compliance with current medications, finances, allergies, liver or kidney disease, and cultural influences.

Apply What You Learned

1. Educational points would include the importance of prescription drugs, various side-effects associated with those drugs, and the importance of telling the physician about the over-the-counter drugs being taken in order to watch for interactions with the prescription drugs.

2. The nurse would point out the medication history to the physician in private prior to the physician going in to assess the client so the appropriate treatment can be prescribed.

3. Over-the-counter drugs are deemed safe by the general public. However, some over-the-counter drugs do not mix well with prescription medications and this client is mixing eight pills, therefore increasing the odds of an adverse reaction. This client should be educated on all of his meds so he can be involved in the treatment plan with his physician and feel some control over his health care plan.

Multiple Choice

1.	C	6.	B	11.	C
2.	D	7.	C	12.	B
3.	A	8.	D	13.	A
4.	A	9.	C	14.	D
5.	B	10.	C	15.	A

Chapter 7 Caring for Clients With Altered Fluid, Electrolyte, or Acid–Base Balance

Key Terms

1.	I	6.	G
2.	H	7.	F
3.	C	8.	J
4.	E	9.	A
5.	D	10.	B

Learning Outcomes

1. ICF is within the cells, accounts for 40% total body weight, and is essential for normal cell function. ECF is outside the cells, accounts for 20% total body weight, and has three compartments: interstitial, intravascular, and transcellular.

2. Water in the body transports nutrients and oxygen to cells, takes waste like carbon dioxide away from the cells, insulates and regulates body temperature, lubricates, and acts as a shock absorber.

3. Electrolytes help regulate water and acid–base balance, contribute to enzyme reactions, and are essential to neuromuscular activity.

4. Components of body fluid regulation are: thirst, kidneys, aldosterone system, antidiuretic hormone, and atrial natriuretic peptide.

5. Sweating, fever, draining wounds, urine, hemorrhage, and GI fluid loss are examples of fluid volume deficits.

6. Renal failure, heart failure, medications, increased sodium intake, and cirrhosis of the liver are some causes of fluid volume excess.

7. Monitoring of fluid status includes serum electrolytes, serum osmolality, hematocrit, urine specific gravity, and central venous pressure.

8. Isotonic solution is used to expand blood volume or replace abnormal loss; hypertonic solution is used to correct sodium depletion, replace water loss, and promote diuresis; and hypotonic solutions are used to maintain sodium and chloride levels as well as to replace water loss.

9. Processed meat and fish, processed grains, canned goods, snack foods, and condiments are examples of high sodium foods.

10. Both hypo- and hyperkalemia affect cardiac function and can result in serious, even fatal, dysrhythmias.

Apply What You Learned

1. The dietician would recommend apricots, bananas, carrots, spinach, meat, fish, and potatoes due to their potassium content.

2. Psychiatry consult based upon the statement regarding solid foods. Ruling out the diagnosis of anorexia nervosa would be necessary.

3. Potassium chloride, because low chloride levels usually accompany low potassium. The physician may or may not order a vitamin supplement depending upon the results of lab tests which will show deficiencies.

Multiple Choice

1. A ✓	6. D	11. A
2. D ✓	7. A	12. A ✓
3. B	8. B	13. D
4. B	9. A ✓	14. B
5. B ✓	10. B ✓	15. C ✓

Chapter 8 Caring for Clients in Pain

Key Terms

1. E ✓	6. I ✓
2. J ✓	7. D ✓
3. H ✓	8. B ✓
4. A ✓	9. C ✓
5. F ✓	10. G ✓

Learning Outcomes

1. Tolerance is the amount and duration of pain a person can stand before seeking relief. Threshold is the point at which each person recognizes pain.

2. Acute pain is temporary, sudden onset and localized. It usually lasts less than six months. Chronic pain is prolonged and lasts longer than six months. It is often unresponsive to conventional medical treatment.

3. Age, sociocultural, emotional status, and past experiences with pain are factors that will affect the client's response to pain.

4. It is a pump with a hand-held button that allows the client to manage their own pain. The dose is programmed into the pump to prevent overdose. It helps the client feel in control of their pain relief.

5. Subjective data would include: location, whether it radiates and where, superficial/deep, onset, pattern, quality, duration, aggravating and relieving factors, intensity, and method of relief.

6. Vital signs, skin moisture and color, dilated pupils, grimacing, guarding, restlessness, moaning, crying, being quiet, and being sad are possible objective indicators of pain.

7. People who ask for opioids are usually addicts. It is best to wait until the client has pain before giving medications, and opioids are too risky to be used in chronic pain.

8. Interventions for pain management include: understanding the client's expectations, including family, using the oral route as this is long-term management, encouraging relaxation or distraction techniques, promoting rest, and proper nutrition, and referring to pain clinic.

9. Complementary therapy includes: acupuncture, biofeedback, relaxation, distraction, hypnotism and cutaneous stimulation.

10. Sedation, respiratory depression, constipation, and nausea are all possible side effects of opioids.

Apply What You Learned

1. The nurse could ask the client how she was directed to take the medication in order to verify that the client understood the directions.

2. The client would have a slow walk, be hunched over, grimacing, holding their back, and possibly moaning and sighing.

3. The client could try deep breathing exercises, relaxation techniques, hypnosis, and distraction such as music.

4. Yes, due to the information given by the client regarding job status and overdue bills. Addiction is also a concern because of the empty medication bottle of 30 pills in only 14 days.

Multiple Choice

1.	A	6.	A	11.	D
2.	D	7.	B	12.	D
3.	A	8.	C	13.	B
4.	B	9.	B	14.	C
5.	C	10.	C	15.	D

Chapter 9 Caring for Clients With Inflammation and Infection

Matching

1. F ✓
2. I ✓
3. G ✓
4. H ✓
5. A ✓

6. E ✓
7. B ✓
8. D ✓
9. J ✓
10. C ✓

Learning Outcomes

1. Inflammation can be caused by mechanical injuries, physical damage such as burns, poisons, bacteria or viruses, extreme heat or cold, hypersensitivity reactions, or by ischemic damage from a stroke or myocardial infarction.

2. There are three steps in the inflammatory response. They are the vascular response, during which blood flow to the injured area increases; cellular response, when white blood cells move into the injured area and ingest harmful bacteria; and healing and tissue repair, when normal structure and function begin to take place.

3. Local inflammation is manifested by redness, warmth, edema, pain, and loss of function.

4. Inflammation that is systemic will present with fever, tachycardia, increased respirations, loss of appetite, fatigue, enlarged lymph nodes, and an elevated white cell count.

5. The chain of infection begins with the microorganism, then proceeds to the reservoir, portal of exit from reservoir, and on to method of transmission. From there it goes to the portal of entry to the susceptible host, and finally to the susceptible host.

6. Chickenpox, gonorrhea, herpes simplex, lyme disease, rabies, tetanus, and tuberculosis are some common infectious diseases.

7. Risk factors for healthcare-associated (nosocomial) infections include: chronic disease, history of frequent antibiotic use, invasive procedures, infections in other sites, burns, length of hospital stay, and the very young or very old age person.

8. Standard precautions involve hand washing, wearing clean gloves, changing gloves between clients, removing soiled clothing as soon as possible, cleaning spills with facility-recommended germicide, and using private rooms when applicable.

9. Fever, sore throat, congestion, runny nose, nausea, weakness, pain on urination, malaise, joint pain, and diarrhea are some subjective data that may be present with the client who has an infection.

10. Objective data for the client with infection would include: vital sign deviations, shortness of breath, altered mental status, dry mucous membranes, wheezes, enlarged lymph nodes, abnormal lab values, and decreased skin turgor.

Apply What You Learned

1. The nurse should expect to see a urinalysis and a white blood cell count with a differential. There may be an order to culture the skin tear.
2. The client does not answer questions appropriately and is confused, so it would be difficult to obtain accurate subjective data.
3. The nurse would expect a broad spectrum antibiotic until test results are evaluated by the physician. There should also be an ointment for the skin tear as well as a dressing to maintain skin integrity and allow healing. Depending upon the facility's policy, a new foley catheter might be placed after the resident is cleansed properly.

Multiple Choice

1. A		6. D		11. D	
2. C		7. D		12. C	
3. B		8. B		13. A	
4. A		9. A		14. B	
5. D		10. C		15. A	

Chapter 10 Caring for Clients Having Surgery

Matching

1. E		6. C
2. J		7. F
3. I		8. B
4. H		9. A
5. G		10. D

Learning Outcomes

1. Inpatient surgery requires admission to a hospital before the procedure, and nursing care in the hospital after the procedure. May be planned or an unanticipated emergency situation. Ambulatory or outpatient surgery is a surgical procedure performed on a client who does not need inpatient nursing care. Procedure can be performed under local or general anesthesia and the client is able to return home without assistance following the procedure.
2. The perioperative nurse must have knowledge of surgical anatomy; anticipate functional disruptions related to surgery; know the potential consequences of disrupted function, risk factors, and potential complications; and understand the emotional and psychosocial effects of surgery on the client and family.
3. Informed consent should include the need for the procedure related to the diagnosis, description and purpose of the procedure, possible benefits and risks, alternative treatments, risks if not done, physician advice to what is needed, and the right to refuse or withdraw the consent.

4. Pre-operative begins when the decision is made and ends when the client is transferred to the operating room. Intra-operative is from when the client enters the operating room and ends in recovery. Post-operative is when the client is in recovery and ends with the client's complete recovery from surgical intervention.

5. The focus of pre-operative care is to obtain informed consent, identify risk factors and needs, physical and psychological preparation of the client, education of the client and family, expected outcomes and recovery.

6. Nursing care on the day of surgery includes the following: verify informed consent, complete skin prep as ordered, ensure ID bands are correct and in place, verify height and weight for anesthesia, remove hair pins and jewelry, obtain vital signs, and provide supportive care to client and family.

7. Anesthesia is the use of chemical substances to produce a loss of sensation, reflex loss, or muscle relaxation during a surgical procedure with or without the loss of consciousness.

8. Risk factors for DVT would include: surgery to lower extremities, varicose veins, over 40 years old, history of emboli, infection, obesity, and malignancy.

9. Dehiscence is a separation of the incision. The wound should be covered immediately with a sterile dressing moistened with normal saline and the surgeon notified. Evisceration is the protrusion of body organs from a wound dehiscence. Cover the wound with a moist sterile dressing or towels and notify the surgeon. Emergency surgery is necessary to repair.

10. PCA pumps allow the client to control and maintain therapeutic blood levels. This method is usually in place for the first few post-operative days and then the client is tapered down to a milder medication such as NSAIDS which act as an adjunct to opioids and are given to treat mild to moderate pain. Pain medications are individually tailored to the client's needs.

Apply What You Learned

1. PCA is a self-administration of opioid medications by a programmed infusion pump. It is utilized in the post-operative period for pain control and allows the client to have some control over their care. It is programmed by the doctors and nurses to ensure safe dosages, and locks out the client once the dosage limit is reached.

2. Research has proven that severe pain is more difficult to treat than pain that is at its onset. Therefore, it is important for the client to notify the nurse once they become uncomfortable in order to treat it effectively. If the pain is controlled, the need for opioids is lessened, or lower dosages will be required. Other pain medications may be utilized instead of an opioid if the client reports pain at its onset.

3. The nurse would ask the client about their expectations toward the pump and treatment, feelings concerning opioid medications like morphine, concerns with addiction, and other methods of pain control. The nurse would also ask the client about their past experiences with pain and how they managed. The client will then feel some sense of control over their care.

Multiple Choice

1. B	6. C	11. C
2. C	7. C	12. B
3. C	8. B	13. B
4. D	9. C	14. C
5. B	10. C	15. C

Chapter 11 Caring for Clients With Altered Immunity

Key Terms

1. E	6. B
2. C	7. J
3. G	8. D
4. A	9. I
5. H	10. F

Learning Outcomes

1. Leukocytes are white blood cells involved in the immune system response. They start in the bone marrow and proceed to attack and destroy any foreign invaders at the site of involvement.

2. The immune system is composed of granulocytes, monocytes, and lymphocytes.

3. IgG is the most abundant in the body and is active against bacteria, toxins, and viruses. It crosses the placenta to provide immune protection to the fetus. The IgA provides local protection to prevent entry of bacteria and viruses, especially through the respiratory and gastrointestinal tracts.

4. Active immunity can be naturally acquired by actually developing the disease or artificially acquired through an immunization. Passive immunity involves injecting serum with ready-made antibodies from other humans or animals.

5. It is recommended that the adult be immunized for MMR, tetanus, Hepatitis B, influenza, and pneumonia.

6. Anaphylaxis is an acute, immediate allergic reaction that requires immediate medical attention.

7. Hypersensitivity reactions can be immediate, cytotoxic, immune, or delayed.

8. Latex can be found in balloons, band-aids, condoms, ace bandages, gloves, wound drains, stethoscopes, urinary catheters, and mattress covers.

9. An autoimmune disorder causes the immune system to mistake itself for nonself, and the body reacts against its own cells. Such disorders are more common in females and the elderly and are frequently associated with a severe physical or psychological stressor.

10. Manifestations of the HIV infection include: fever, sore throat, headache, rash, fatigue, night sweats, weight loss, diarrhea, wasting syndrome, toxoplasmosis, herpes simplex/zoster, Kaposi's sarcoma, and Non-Hodgkin's lymphoma.

Apply What You Learned

1. The nurse would explain that KS is the most common cancer associated with HIV infection. Tumors develop in the lining of the small blood vessels that cause the lesions on the skin. They start out painless but may become painful as the disease progresses.
2. The white patches in the mouth of this client are called oral candidiasis or thrush. It is a fungal infection and may extend into the esophagus and stomach. It can produce an unpleasant taste in the mouth and can lead to painful swallowing.
3. Provide continuity of care and support to the client and his partner. Balance activity with rest periods, provide a quiet room with minimal lighting, encourage socialization and pleasant conversation, focus on the things the client can do and praise for when tasks are accomplished, provide distractions such as music, television, or movies.

Multiple Choice

1. C
2. C
3. D
4. D
5. A

6. A
7. C
8. C
9. C
10. A

11. B
12. B
13. B
14. C
15. C

Chapter 12 Caring for Clients With Cancer

Key Terms

1. E
2. D
3. G
4. A
5. C

6. B
7. F
8. J
9. H
10. I

Learning Outcomes

1. Benign neoplasms are localized growths with well-defined borders, and are usually encapsulated. They tend to respond to body controls, and once removed rarely recur. Malignant neoplasms grow aggressively and do not respond to the body controls. They are not easy to remove and can recur. When the term cancer is used, it is referring to a malignant tumor.
2. An oncogene is a gene capable of promoting uncontrolled cellular growth. Carcinogens can "activate" the oncogene, thus allowing tumor development.
3. Controllable risk factors associated with cancer include stress, diet, weight, occupation, tobacco use, alcohol and drug use, and sun exposure.

4. HIV, Hepatitis B, arsenic, asbestos, ultraviolet rays, radon, cigarettes, and hormones like estrogen are some carcinogens associated with cancer.
5. Possible cancer warning signs include: persistent cough or hoarseness; unusual bleeding or discharge; recent unintended weight loss; recent change in a wart, mole, skin color, or texture; persistent functional change such as SOB; or a palpable lump in tissue.
6. There are many common manifestations regarding cancer. Pain, anemia, fatigue, bruising, anorexia, hoarseness, jaundice, constipation, and mental status changes, as well as difficulty swallowing, can be indicators of the disease.
7. Anorexia-cachexia syndrome is the effect of cancer cells on metabolism; cancer cells divert nutrition to their own use, inhibit food intake, and break down body tissue and muscle proteins to support their growth.
8. Tumor classification system begins with the name of origin. It proceeds to grading where the aggressiveness is described. Staging is the last component and this refers to the relative size of the tumor and extent of the disease.
9. Superior Vena Cava syndrome, pericardial effusion, sepsis, spinal cord compression, and tumor lysis syndrome are oncologic emergencies.
10. Common side effects resulting from chemotherapy are: bone marrow suppression, nausea, vomiting, diarrhea, stomatitis, alopecia, and lethargy.

Apply What You Learned

1. The nurse could encourage the client to eat whatever is appealing in order to maintain caloric intake, even if it is not nutritionally sound. Encourage the intake of small, frequent meals with the use of an antiemetic. Nutritional supplements could be suggested, along with keeping a food diary to validate intake.
2. The nurse should begin by creating an open environment for the client and family to discuss feelings realistically. Answer all questions honestly and encourage the client to continue to take part in activities they enjoy.
3. Hospice care allows the client to elect to die at home or in a home-like setting. The hospice nurse is usually on call 24-hours a day and attends the client often. The nurse continually assesses the comfort of the client to ensure they have as much pain control as possible. The nurse is often with the family when the client dies. The support from hospice is for the entire family, not just the client.

Multiple Choice

1.	C	6.	A	11.	A
2.	C	7.	C	12.	D
3.	B	8.	C	13.	B
4.	D	9.	D	14.	B
5.	B	10.	A	15.	A

Chapter 13 Loss, Grief, and End-of-Life Care

Matching

1. H ✓
2. E ✓
3. A ✓
4. C ✓
5. G ✓

6. B ✓
7. D ✓
8. F ✓
9. I ✓
10. J ✓

Learning Outcomes

1. Grief is the emotional response to loss and its accompanying changes. Whereas loss occurs when a valued object, person, body part, or situation that was formerly present is lost or changed and can no longer be seen, felt, heard, known, or experienced.

2. Kubler-Ross identified the following stages of grief: Denial, Anger, Bargaining, Depression, and Acceptance. She observed that not all people will go through the stages in order and some may linger at a particular stage until they are ready to move on to the next stage. This staging process is individualized based upon the person's response to the loss.

3. Health, social status, possessions, lifestyle, sexual functioning, body parts, death, marital relationships, and reproduction are some common fears of loss.

4. Advance Directives can be presented as a living will, health care surrogate, or as a durable power of attorney.

5. DNR, or no code, is written by the physician for the client who is near death. This order is usually based on the wishes of the client and family that no CPR be performed for respiratory or cardiac arrest. A comfort-measures-only order indicates that no further life-sustaining interventions are necessary and that the goal of care is a comfortable, dignified death.

6. Euthanasia is a term that is used to signify a killing that is prompted by some humanitarian motive, for example, in a stage IV cancer patient who has uncontrolled pain and is cognitively aware of the pain.

7. Manifestations of impending death are: difficulty talking or swallowing, nausea or abdominal distension, urinary incontinence, constipation, decreased senses, weak or irregular pulse, decreasing blood pressure, decreased respirations, changes in level of consciousness, restlessness, and cyanosis of the extremities.

8. To maintain comfort of the dying client, the nurse should maintain clean skin and bed linens. A draw sheet should be used to turn the client frequently and comfortably. Gentle massage to promote circulation shift edema as tolerated by the client. Provide small, frequent sips of liquids. Provide oral care and clean secretions from eyes and nose. Administer ordered pain medication and oxygen.

9. Hospice care is for clients and their families when faced with a limited life expectancy. It is initiated for clients as they near the end of life and emphasizes quality rather than quantity of life.

10. Indications that death has occurred include: absent respiration, pulse, and heartbeat; fixed, dilated pupils; release of stool and urine; pallor and waxen color; drop in body temperature; lack of reflexes; and flat encephalogram.

Apply What You Learned

1. The type of care that this client is to receive is termed hospice. It focuses on the quality of life that is left, not the quantity. The goal is to ensure a comfortable and dignified passing.
2. When explaining procedures to this client, the nurse needs to use short sentences, speak calmly yet loudly enough for them to hear, demonstrate by using touch in a sensitive and caring manner, and allow the client to participate as much as possible. The nurse needs to ensure proper rest periods are offered during care as the client may tire easily.
3. The nurse would explain to the family that their loved one may not take in any more oral fluids or food items as the dying process begins. The client may become agitated and this is common. The family needs the reassurance to not take this personally. Bowel and bladder incontinence is a common manifestation and the staff will do everything possible to maintain clean and dry skin. The family will see skin color changes as the body proceeds in death. Vital signs will become irregular and the level of consciousness will change. Aside from these findings, the nurse needs to be empathetic and open with the family. They will be looking to the nurse for emotional support during this confusing and difficult time.

Multiple Choice

1. B
2. D
3. A
4. A
5. C
6. C
7. B
8. C
9. B
10. C
11. B
12. C
13. B
14. A
15. B

Chapter 14 Caring for Clients Experiencing Shock, Trauma, or Disasters

Matching

1. H
2. I
3. J
4. G
5. D
6. E
7. F
8. B
9. A
10. C

Learning Outcomes

1. Shock is a life-threatening condition, characterized by inadequate blood flow to the tissues and cells.
2. The five types of shock are: hypovolemic, anaphylactic, cardiogenic, septic, and neurogenic.
3. Compensated, progressive, and irreversible are the three stages of shock.
4. Anaphylactic shock presents itself with the client having difficulty breathing, tachycardic, hypotensive, restless, and a decreased level of consciousness.

5. An autotransfusion is the collection, filtration, and retransfusion of a client's own blood. Blood from the chest cavity is the typical source for an autotransfusion.

6. Blood and blood products are represented by: whole blood, packed red cells, platelets, fresh frozen plasma, and cryoprecipitate.

7. Nursing implications for blood transfusions may be basic, but extremely important. Vital signs need to obtained prior to transfusion so there is a baseline record. The nurse must stay with the client for the first 15 minutes of the transfusion to monitor for adverse reactions. Take and record vital signs during the transfusion as facility policy indicates. If a reaction occurs, stop the infusion and begin a drip of normal saline and follow facility policy.

8. Trauma is an injury caused by physical force and is the number one cause of death for persons under the age of 35.

9. Blunt trauma does not cause a break in the skin and can result in greater internal damage than what appears on the surface. Whereas a penetrating trauma results from foreign objects that pierce the body. Again, the external appearance does not determine the extent of internal damage.

10. To be safe in your home, use nonskid mats in the shower, install handrails by the tub and toilet as needed, use night-lights, turn pot handles away from the edge of the stove, keep a fire extinguisher near the stove, remove clutter from pathways, keep stairs well lit, install smoke alarms, and keep firearms locked.

Apply What You Learned

1. This would be classified as a blunt trauma injury because there is no break in the skin.

2. The nurse would ask what time the injury occurred, how fast was the ball going, where exactly on the head he was hit, did he lose consciousness, did he vomit, how is his vision now and how was it then, pain scale, radiating pain, stiffness in the neck, past traumas to the head, complaints of dizziness and allergies. This information would help the nurse decide the urgency of the injury.

3. Radiography studies would be completed and could include CT scans, MRIs and nuclear medicine. These studies would verify breaks, fractures, and fluid on the brain. Labs would also be drawn to check inflammatory response markers and to have a baseline should the client experience complications. For treatment, the nurse would expect to provide a quiet and dimly lit room, ice packs for the first 24-hour period, pain medication as needed, neuro exam completed by the physician with follow-up by the nurse and monitoring for nausea, vomiting, level of consciousness, and pain.

Multiple Choice

1. D
2. B
3. A
4. D
5. C

6. B
7. A
8. A
9. B
10. A

11. B
12. D
13. B
14. C
15. D

Chapter 15 The Cardiovascular System and Assessment

Matching

1. A
2. E
3. F
4. I
5. C

6. G
7. J
8. H
9. D
10. B

Learning Outcomes

1. The heart is a hollow, cone-shaped organ approximately the size of an adult's fist which weighs less than one pound. It is located behind the sternum and between the lungs in the thoracic cavity, slightly to the left of midline. The heart is a double pump. The right side receives blood from the body and pumps it to the lungs, and the left side receives blood from the lungs and pumps it to the body.
2. Diastole is when the ventricles fill and are relaxed. Systole is when the ventricles contract and eject blood into the pulmonary and systemic circuits.
3. The peripheral vascular system is a network of blood vessels that carry blood to peripheral tissues and then return it to the heart. This network includes arteries, veins, and capillaries.
4. Electrocardiogram is a record of the heart's electrical activity detected by electrodes placed on the skin. Patterns are used to detect dysrhythmias, myocardial damage or enlargement, and the effects of drugs.
5. Contractility is the natural ability of the cardiac muscle fibers to shorten during systole. It is necessary to move blood into circulation.
6. Cardiac output is the amount of blood pumped by the ventricles in one minute. It indicates how well the heart is functioning. The average adult cardiac output ranges from 4–8 liters per minute.
7. Activity level, autonomic nervous system, and hormones affect the heart rate.
8. Components of a lipid profile include: total cholesterol, triglycerides, high-density lipoproteins, low-density lipoproteins, and very low-density lipoproteins.
9. Doppler studies, transthoracic echocardiogram, stress tests, CXR, angiography, cardiac catheterization, CT, MRI, and radionuclear scans are used as diagnostic tools in cardiac dysfunction.
10. The purpose of a cardiac MRI is to show the thickness of the heart walls, size of the chambers, valve function, and coronary vessel flow.

Apply What You Learned

1. Complete only a brief, focused assessments on the acute symptoms. Notify charge nurse and physician. Complete assessment data collection once the acute symptoms have been relieved and the client is resting comfortably.
2. Diagnostic testing includes: lipid profile, C-reactive protein, serum cardiac markers, cardiac hormones, 12-lead ECG, telemetry monitoring, and imaging studies.

Multiple Choice

1.	A	6.	C	11.	B
2.	C	7.	A	12.	A
3.	C	8.	A	13.	B
4.	B	9.	D	14.	A
5.	D	10.	D	15.	B

Chapter 16 Caring for Clients With Coronary Heart Disease and Dysrhythmias

Matching

1.	C	6.	B
2.	G	7.	F
3.	I	8.	D
4.	A	9.	J
5.	E	10.	H

Learning Outcomes

1. Modifiable risk factors are: hypertension, smoking, diabetes, obesity, inactivity, and a diet high in saturated fats. Non-modifiable risk factors are: age, gender, race, and heredity.
2. Atherosclerosis is a disease in which lesions (plaque) develop in the lining of the medium and large arteries. They protrude into the artery and may affect blood flow through the artery. It is the primary cause of coronary heart disease.
3. Manifestations of angina include: chest pain that may radiate to the neck, arms, shoulders, or jaw along with tight, squeezing, or heavy chest pain. The client may experience chest pain brought on by exercise, strong emotion, stress, cold, and heavy meals. The client with angina also may have shortness of breath, pallor, anxiety, and fear.
4. Manifestations of an acute myocardial infarction include: chest pain, tachycardia, shortness of breath, cool and clammy skin, diaphoresis, anxiety, feeling of impending doom, and nausea and vomiting.
5. Cardiac dysrhythmias are disturbances or irregularities in the electrical system of the heart. They can be benign or life-threatening.
6. Cardioversion, also known as defibrillation, is used to treat rhythms that affect cardiac output and the client's welfare. An electrical shock is administered to depolarize all cells of the heart at the same time. This often stops the abnormal rhythm and allows the sinus node to resume control of the rhythm.
7. Sudden cardiac death is when death occurs within one hour of the onset of cardiac symptoms.
8. Calan, Isoptin, Cardizem, and Dilacor are calcium channel blockers.
9. PVCs are ectopic ventricular beats that occur before the next expected beat of the normal rhythm. They may be isolated or occur in patterns.
10. Atrial flutter is a very rapid and regular atrial rhythm. The client usually complains of palpitations or a fluttering in the chest or throat.

Apply What You Learned

1. The nurse needs to instruct the client about pain management after the procedure. Movement of the affected arm and shoulder will be restricted for the first 24 hours. A chest x-ray will be done post procedure for placement verification. The client will receive a card with the pacemaker's name, model number, rate, and battery life. They need to carry this card at all times and should wear a Medic-Alert bracelet. Teach the client about the function of the pacemaker and how to take and record their pulse rate.
2. Decreased Cardiac Output, Risk for Ineffective Cardiac Tissue Perfusion, and Anxiety are nursing diagnoses related to this client.
3. The client should call his physician when the pulse rate is 5 or more bpm slower than the preset pacemaker rate, or if they experience fever, dizziness, fainting, fatigue, weakness, chest pain, or palpitations. All of the client's providers must be aware that the client has a pacemaker implanted.

Multiple Choice

1.	B	6.	D	11.	C
2.	C	7.	B	12.	D
3.	B	8.	A	13.	B
4.	C	9.	B	14.	B
5.	D	10.	B	15.	C

Chapter 17 Caring for Clients With Cardiac Disorders

Matching

1.	I	6.	C
2.	E	7.	F
3.	G	8.	A
4.	B	9.	H
5.	J	10.	D

Learning Outcomes

1. Heart failure is the inability of the heart to function as a pump to meet the needs of the body.
2. Teaching points for the older adult include: Longer warm-up and cool-down with exercise, engage in regular exercise 3–4 times a week, rest with feet elevated, maintain adequate fluid intake, and reduce sodium intake in diet.
3. A: high risk for heart failure but no current structural or functional damage, B: structual heart disease with no symptoms of heart failure, C: structural heart disease with current or prior symptoms of heart failure, and D: advanced heart disease with symptoms of heart failure at rest despite treatment.
4. Rheumatic fever is a systemic inflammatory disease caused by an abnormal immune response to infection by group A beta-hemolytic streptococci.

5. Fever, joint pain, inflammation, rash on trunk, chest pain, tachycardia, shortness of breath, cardiac friction rub, possible murmur, and involuntary muscle spasms are manifestations of rheumatic fever.
6. People with rheumatic heart disease, prosthetic heart valves, previous endocarditis, congenital heart conditions, and mitral valve prolapse should receive prophylactic antibiotics.
7. Pericarditis is inflammation of the preicardium, the outermost layer of the heart.
8. The types of heart murmurs are: mitral stenosis, mitral regurgitation, aortic stenosis, and aortic regurgitation.
9. Cardiomyopathy is a disorder that affects the structure and function of the heart muscle.
10. MVP is a form of mitral insufficiency that occurs when the posterior cusp of the mitral valve flops back into the left atrium during systole. Most clients with MVP are asymptomatic and it is usually congenital in nature. It is commonly found in young women between the ages of 14 and 30 and its incidence declines with age.

Apply What You Learned

1. This client will have vital sign monitoring, neck vein distention and level of consciousness assessments, intake and output measurements, fluid restriction as ordered by physician, oxygen and pulse oximetry, medications as ordered and physical, emotional, and mental rest should be promoted.
2. The nurse would contact the dietician for a heart healthy diet and a social worker to assist in finding either home health care or a rehab facility where the client can go until he is strong enough to manage on his own.
3. The nurse would teach the client how to take his pulse before and after activities. The client should also be encourage to gradually increase activity and self-care as tolerated. The client should be encouraged to ask for help when necessary because energy-saving techniques reduce cardiac workload.

Multiple Choice

1.	C	6.	D	11.	A
2.	C	7.	C	12.	B
3.	A	8.	B	13.	B
4.	B	9.	A	14.	C
5.	B	10.	C	15.	B

Chapter 18 Caring for Clients With Peripheral Vascular Disorders

Matching

1.	E	6.	I
2.	F	7.	H
3.	D	8.	G
4.	C	9.	J
5.	A	10.	B

Learning Outcomes

1. Hypertension is defined as a blood pressure higher than 140mm Hg systolic or 90 mm Hg diastolic on three separate readings several weeks apart.
2. Risk factors for hypertension include: obesity, insulin resistance, excess alcohol consumption, smoking, physical stress, family history, age, and race.
3. Abdominal aortic aneurysms present with abdominal pain, lower back pain, cool and pale lower extremities, and a pulsating abdominal mass.
4. Marfan syndrome is a connective tissue disorder with three distinctive features: Long, thin extremities, hyperextensible joints and other skeletal deformities; impaired vision; and cardiovascular defects including MVP and weakness of the aorta. There is no cure for Marfan syndrome.
5. Arteriosclerosis is a common arterial disorder characterized by thickening, loss of elasticity, and calcification of arterial walls.
6. Complementary therapies for PVD include: aromatherapy, healing touch, imagery, magnets, massage, yoga, breathing exercises, and counseling.
7. Raynaud's phenomenon is characterized by spasms of the small arteries and arterioles of the extremities. It is often secondary to another disorder, and is sometimes called the red-white-and-blue disease. The spasms cause the fingers to go blue and white, and then to red when the spasm is close to ending.
8. Risk factors for venous thrombosis include: previous episodes, prolonged immobility, major surgery, myocardial infarction, certain cancers, pregnancy, or childbirth, estrogen therapy, and obesity.
9. Varicose veins are irregular, tortuous veins with poorly functioning valves. They commonly affect the lower extremities.
10. Manifestations of varicose veins include: severe, aching, leg pain; leg heaviness; itching of the leg; heat in the leg after prolonged standing, and visibly dilated veins in the leg.

Apply What You Learned

1. The diagnosis most likely in this case is Raynaud's phenomenon.
2. Treatments for this disease include: smoking cessation, regular exercise, keeping the extremeties warm by wearing gloves and trying to avoid injury to the hands. Amputation is only done if blood flow can not be restored and tissue necrosis has occurred.

Multiple Choice

1.	A	6.	B	11.	A
2.	C	7.	C	12.	A
3.	C	8.	D	13.	A
4.	D	9.	B	14.	D
5.	C	10.	A	15.	B

Matching

1.	C	6.	J
2.	F	7.	H
3.	G	8.	E
4.	B	9.	I
5.	D	10.	A

Learning Outcomes

1. Plasma is a clear yellow, protein-rich fluid in which the red cells, white cells, and platelets are suspended.
2. Hemoglobin is an oxygen-carrying protein which contains iron. This iron binds with oxygen and is synthesized within the RBC.
3. The differential includes: neutrophils, eosinophils, basophils, lymphocytes, and monocytes.
4. Platelets are an essential part of the body's clotting mechanism. They are small fragments of cytoplasm without nuclei that contain many granules. They are stored in the spleen before being release into circulation. They live approximately ten days in circulating blood.
5. The lymphatic system assists the immune system by removing foreign matter, infectious organisms, and tumor cells from lymph. The largest lymphoid organ is the spleen and it filters the blood and produces lymphocytes and stores blood and platelets.
6. Lab tests used in lymphatic disorders are: CBC, clotting studies, Coombs' test, hemoglobin electrophoresis, iron studies, and Schilling's test.
7. A bone marrow aspiration is done to analyze bone marrow and establish a diagnosis. Marrow is obtained from the posterior superior iliac crest and may be painful for the client despite the use of local anesthesia. The biopsy is done to examine for presence of abnormal cells.
8. The five stages of hemostasis are: vessel spasms, formation of the platelet plug, clot formation, clot retraction, and clot dissolution.
9. Blood transports oxygen and nutrients to cells, essential substances to cells, and tissues and waste products away from tissues for removal from the body.
10. Normal hemoglobin for men is 14–16.5 g/dLl and 12–15 g/dLl in women.

Apply What You Learned

1. Aside from a CBC to include a WBC with differential, the nurse should expect a bone marrow aspiration to rule out malignancy.
2. Regarding the bone marrow aspiration, the client should be informed that the procedure takes about 20 minutes. A local anesthetic will be used but they may still feel some pressure with the procedure. It is important to remain very still during the procedure and the site may ache for several days. The client should be taught to report any unusual bleeding, drainage, or symptoms of infection immediately.

Multiple Choice

1.	C	6.	B	11.	A
2.	C	7.	B	12.	B
3.	D	8.	A	13.	C
4.	A	9.	C	14.	A
5.	A	10.	D	15.	A

Chapter 20 Caring for Clients With Hematologic and Lymphatic Disorders

Matching

1.	C	6.	D
2.	H	7.	A
3.	I	8.	J
4.	B	9.	F
5.	G	10.	E

Learning Outcomes

1. Anemia is a condition in which the hemoglobin concentration, or the number of circulating RBCs, is decreased.
2. Thalassemia is an inherited disorder also caused by abnormal hemoglobin synthesis. It commonly affects people of Mediterranean, Asian, or African descent. The client may have few symptoms or severe disease depending on the form of the disorder.
3. Asparagus, spinach, broccoli, green beans, corn flakes, oatmeal, and pasta contain folic acid.
4. Polycythemia is an abnormally high red blood cell count with high hematocrit.
5. Manifestations of leukemia include: anemia, fatigue, tachycardia, malaise, lethargy, and dyspnea. The client may also present with headache, altered level of consciousness, edema, anorexia, nausea, and bruising.
6. Acute myeloid, chronic myeloid, acute lymphocytic, and chronic lymphocytic are the four types of leukemia.
7. Nursing diagnoses with leukemia include: Risk for Infection, Impaired Oral Mucous Membranes, and Grieving.
8. Agranulocytosis is a decrease in granulocytes. Impaired WBC formation in the bone marrow is the usual cause.
9. Thrombocytopenia is a platelet count of less than 100,000 platelets per milliliter of blood. It is the most common cause of abnormal bleeding. It typically affects young adults from ages 20–40, and women more than men.
10. Risk factors associated with DIC are: infection, malignancy, trauma, liver disease, hematologic disorders, venomous snakebites, and acute respiratory distress syndrome.

Apply What You Learned

1. Hodgkin's disease would be the diagnosis.
2. Chemotherapy and radiation are the treatments of choice for this disease.
3. Nursing diagnoses for this disorder include: Risk for Impaired Skin Integrity, Nausea, Fatigue, and Disturbed Body Image.

Multiple Choice

1. A	6. C	11. A
2. D	7. B	12. C
3. D	8. B	13. C
4. C	9. A	14. C
5. C	10. D	15. A

Chapter 21 The Respiratory System and Assessment

Matching

1. B	6. A	
2. I	7. E	
3. H	8. F	
4. D	9. C	
5. J	10. G	

Learning Outcomes

1. The function of the upper respiratory system is to clean, humidify, and warm air. An open upper airway is needed for effective breathing.
2. The nose, sinuses, pharynx, and larynx are structures of the upper respiratory system.
3. The function of the lower respiratory system is to provide oxygen to the cells of the body and to eliminate carbon dioxide, a waste product of metabolism.
4. The lungs, bronchi, and alveoli are structures of the lower respiratory system.
5. Age-related changes in the respiratory system include: decreased mobility of the rib cage, anterior-posterior diameter decrease, muscles of respiration weaken, and the cough and laryngeal reflexes are less effective.
6. Adventitious breath sounds are lung sounds that are abnormal.
7. Pulse oximetry is a non-invasive test used to evaluate and monitor oxygen saturation. The normal range is 95% or higher. The pulse oximeter sensor is usually applied to a fingertip and the sensor emits infrared light to evaluate the oxygen saturation percentage. Infrared light is absorbed by hemoglobin.
8. In obtaining a throat swab, use a sterile cotton swab or throat swab kit. Identify the client and purpose of the procedure and provide privacy. Have the client in the seated position, if possible. Use standard precautions. Have the client open their mouth, extend tongue and say "ah." Quickly swab the tonsils, any exudate, and any red areas. Insert the swab into the specimen container and avoid contamination. Make sure to label the container and send to the laboratory.

9. The VP scan is used to detect pulmonary emboli, evaluate chronic lung disease and assess the function of lung transplants.

10. Inform the family and the client that the procedure takes 30–45 minutes. It may be done in the operating room, client room or a procedure room. The client will receive an anesthetic and will have little discomfort. The client may have a sore throat and hoarse voice following the procedure. The client may have a fever for the first 24 hours after as well. They must report persistent cough, bloody sputum, wheezing, shortness of breath, or chest pain to their doctor.

Apply What You Learned

1. This client will need a focused assessment on the respiratory system. Listening to the lungs in the front and the back will be important observations for the nurse.

2. Diagnostic testing the nurse might see include: pulmonary function test (PFT), CBC, chemistries, throat cultures, and chest x-rays.

3. The nurse needs to ask the client if there are factors that precipitate the symptoms and what alleviates them. The nurse should ask for remedies he may have tried at home along with asking what allergies he has. The nurse should also find out if the client has traveled anywhere out of his region or has been exposed to something different in his environment.

Multiple Choice

1. B	6. A	11. A
2. A	7. C	12. B
3. D	8. D	13. A
4. C	9. C	14. C
5. C	10. C	15. A

Chapter 22 Caring for Clients With Upper Respiratory Disorders

Matching

1. D	6. A
2. B	7. G
3. E	8. C
4. I	9. H
5. F	10. J

Learning Outcomes

1. Viral pharyngitis is manifested through low grade fevers, sore throat, headache, and has a gradual onset. Streptococcal will have a fever higher than 102, severe sore throat, patches on tonsils, malaise, and dysphagia.

2. Rhinitis is an inflammation of the nasal cavity and is the most common upper respiratory disorder. Sinusitis is an inflammation of the mucous membranes of the sinuses and often follows a URI.

3. People over 50, nursing home residents, pregnant women, those with chronic disorders, healthcare workers, and family of at-risk clients should receive the influenza vaccine.

4. To control URIs in LTC: discourage people who are ill from visiting, provide tissues and masks to residents and visitors with symptoms, provide hand sanitizer and handwashing supplies, ensure healthcare staff knows standard precautions, move residents with influenza symptoms to private rooms and provide annual influenza vaccines to residents and staff.

5. Stridor is a high-pitched, harsh sound heard during inspiration.

6. Ineffective Breathing Pattern, Ineffective Airway Clearance, and Disturbed Sleep Pattern are some nursing diagnoses for clients with URIs.

7. Also known as whooping cough, pertussis is an acute, highly contagious URI. Teens have the highest incidence but it also affects adults and young children. It is a reportable disease to local county health departments. Household contact of the infected person should take prophylactic antibiotics.

8. Epistaxis is nosebleed caused by picking, injury, dryness, infection or substance abuse.

9. Manifestations of nasal fractures include: epistaxis, deformity or displacement, crepitus, soft tissue trauma, and instability of the nasal bridge.

10. The temporary absence of breathing during sleep. Affects men more than women. Obesity, enlarged tonsils, and the use of ETOH and sedatives before sleep contribute to sleep apnea. Obstructive sleep apnea is the most common form. It occurs when the pharynx is obstructed by the soft palate and tongue.

Apply What You Learned

1. The nurse would tell the client that his quality of life will be better if he were to quit drinking and smoking. Also, the healing process after surgery will be improved and the risk of infection will be reduced as well. This client may benefit from a support group such as A.A. or a psychologist to assist with the issue of terminal illness.

2. Encourage the family to visit whenever possible. Discuss postoperative communication techniques because this surgery will result in a loss of speech and the client will breathe through a permanent stoma in the neck. Teach the client to cough and deep breathe effectively and to support the head when moving in bed. The client and family should be taught how to protect the stoma from particulate matter in the air with gauze or other stoma protector. Encourage the client and family to express their fears and anxieties.

3. Postoperatively, the nurse will be monitoring the respiratory status, oxygen saturation, and maintaining humidified oxygen. The nurse will suction the tracheostomy using sterile technique as needed and provide care per protocol. The client will be maintained on intravenous fluids and/or enteral feeding until able to take adequate amounts of food and fluids orally.

Multiple Choice

1. C	6. D	11. B
2. B	7. B	12. B
3. B	8. C	13. D
4. C	9. C	14. C
5. C	10. D	15. B

Chapter 23 Caring for Clients With Lower Respiratory Disorders

Matching

1. C	6. E
2. H	7. D
3. F	8. A
4. J	9. B
5. G	10. I

Learning Outcomes

1. Dyspnea is difficulty breathing, hemoptysis is bloody sputum, and cyanosis is a bluish-gray skin color.

2. Aspiration of gastric contents into the lungs causes a chemical and bacterial pneumonia. The risk for aspiration pneumonia is highest during emergency surgery and when cough and gag reflexes are depressed or swallowing is impaired.

3. Sputum gram stain and culture and sensitivity, CBC, WBC with differential, ABGs, pulse oximetry, chest x-ray, and bronchoscopy are some diagnostic testing to be done for pneumonia.

4. Ineffective Airway Clearance, Ineffective Breathing Pattern, and Activity Intolerance are nursing diagnoses for pneumonia.

5. TB is a chronic, recurrent infectious disease that usually affects the lungs. It can also involve other organs. Clients will present with fatigue, weight loss, anorexia, low-grade afternoon fever and night sweats. The cough is dry intially and later becomes productive of purulent or blood-tinged sputum. This is when the client usually seeks medical attention.

6. Less than 5 mm induration is negative for TB. Greater than 15 mm induration is positive for TB in all people while 5–15mm induration can be positive for people with certain illnesses or risk factors.

7. Asthma is chronic inflammatory disorder of the airways characterized by recurrent episodes of wheezing, breathlessness, chest tightness, and coughing.

8. Manifestations of COPD include: Productive cough, dyspnea, exercise tolerance for as long as ten years, cough usually in the morning (smokers' cough), episodes of increased sputum and difficulty breathing are common and often caused by respiratory infections.

9. Anterior–posterior chest diameter increases, taking on the appearaance of a barrel. This occurs from the alveoli becoming less elastic and airways tend to collapse during exhalation. This causes air trapping in the lungs.

10. Lung cancer presents with: cough, hemoptysis, wheeze, chest pain, weight loss, fever, fluid and electrolyte imbalance, anemia, and peripheral neuropathy.

Apply What You Learned

1. The client will receive local anesthetic and may feel pressure upon insertion. Her breathing will improve once inserted. The nurse will document vital signs, breath sounds, saturation, color, and respiratory effort at least every four hours. The collection device will be kept below chest level and upright to maintain seal. The nurse will measure the drainage every eight hours and report to the physician. If the tube is removed accidentally, the nurse will immediately apply a sterile, occlusive dressing and notify the physician.

2. Impaired Gas Exchange and Risk for Injury are nursing diagnoses that apply to this client with chest tubes.

3. The nurse will frequently evaluate the respiratory status and oxygenation along with the amount of drainage and functioning of the drainage system. The nurse will document all teaching provided, including a smoking cessation program. The nurse will also document the client's tolerance to ADL, intake, output, and ambulation efforts.

Multiple Choice

1. D
2. D
3. C
4. C
5. D

6. D
7. D
8. D
9. B
10. A

11. A
12. A
13. C
14. C
15. A

Chapter 24 The Gastrointestinal System and Assessment

Matching

1. E
2. I
3. F
4. J
5. H

6. D
7. A
8. C
9. G
10. B

Learning Outcomes

1. Peristalsis is the alternating waves of contraction and relaxation. These waves keep food moving through the GI tract.

2. The GI tract includes the mouth, pharynx, esophagus, stomach, small intestine, and large intestine.

3. The liver metabolizes carbohydrates, proteins, and fats. It eliminates old blood cells, cellular debris, and bacteria. The liver also stores blood, vitamins, and minerals, and excretes bile.

4. An upper endoscopy is used to evaluate swallowing problems, gastric reflux, and peptic ulcer disease.

5. The images can alert the physician to any obstruction or tumor that may be present.

6. Esophageal manometry measures the pressure of the esophageal sphincters and peristalsis. This tool can be helpful when the physician suspects swallowing dysfunction.

7. Liver, gallbladder, pylorus, duodenum, right adrenal gland, and a portion of the right kidney are located in the right upper quadrant of the abdomen.

8. The purpose of the stool specimen test for ova and parasites is to detect the presence of infective organisms.

9. When deficient in vitamins and minerals, the skin may be dry, flaky, and bruise easily. The client may also have joint pain and peripheral neuropathies.

10. Weakness, weight loss, and increased heart rate are associated with water deficit. While increased blood pressure, weight gain, edema, and shortness of breath are indicators of water excess.

Apply What You Learned

1. The nurse should ask the client about recent lifestyle changes and weight loss. Find out if the client has traveled out of the region or has noticed blood in his stool. The nurse should also find out what the pain is relieved by, exacerbated by, and if it radiates. The nurse should try to do a diet recall with the client and explore what he has been eating over this time period.

2. The nurse would begin the assessment of the abdomen with the inspection of the area, followed by auscultation. Never palpate an abdomen without listening for bowel sounds first.

3. A CT scan will be done to rule out obstruction, along with a flat plate x-ray of the abdomen. Depending upon the results, the physician may order a barium enema or an upper endoscopy.

4. This client should be NPO until diagnostic testing is complete and read by the physician.

Multiple Choice

1.	A	6.	D	11.	D
2.	C	7.	C	12.	B
3.	B	8.	C	13.	C
4.	B	9.	D	14.	C
5.	D	10.	A	15.	B

Matching

1.	J	6.	H
2.	C	7.	A
3.	F	8.	B
4.	E	9.	D
5.	G	10.	I

Learning Outcomes

1. Obesity is an excess of adipose tissue and occurs when excess calories are stored as fat. Morbid obesity is body weight of more than 100% over ideal weight.
2. Heart failure, hypertension, osteoarthritis, cancer, and muscle strains are some complications related to obesity.
3. Behavior strategies for weight loss include: controlling the environment, controlling physical responses to food, controlling psychosocial responses to food, and making exercise a daily routine.
4. Aging, AIDS, burns, cancer, eating disorders, and surgery are conditions that are associated with malnutrition.
5. Catabolism is the breakdown of cells and tissues.
6. Enteral feedings may be used to meet all or part of the nutritional needs in clients who are unable to eat. Enteral feedings are done through various types of tubes that go directly into the GI tract via the nose, stomach, or jejunum.
7. Anorexia nervosa is an intense fear of weight gain and weight less than 85% of expected for age and height.
8. Stomatitis is inflammation of the oral mucosa that affects eating.
9. Oral cancer can be a product of a sore in the mouth that does not heal. It can also manifest as irregular white patches on the lips or tongue, or through difficult swallowing and a sore throat.
10. GERD is the backward movement of gastric contents into the esophagus. It affects 15–20% of adults and is considered to be a common GI disorder.

Apply What You Learned

1. The client must be prepared for a complete change in lifestyle with regards to dietary habits in order for the surgery to be successful. A strict diet will need to be followed for the rest of the client's life to prevent weight gain and complications. The nurse must question the client's readiness for the long-term behavioral changes that will accompany this procedure. The surgeon will then clarify the importance of following the diet again, before obtaining the consent.
2. The client needs to be instructed on the signs and symptoms of infection, dumping syndrome, postprandial hypoglycemia, and pernicious anemia.
3. Pain, airway monitoring, infection monitoring, imbalanced nutrition, and accurate intake and output would be priorities regarding this client.

Multiple Choice

1.	C ✓	6.	B ✓	11.	C
2.	D ✓	7.	C	12.	C
3.	B ✓	8.	C ✓	13.	B
4.	B ✓	9.	B ✓	14.	B ✓
5.	C	10.	A ✓	15.	D

Chapter 26 Caring for Clients With Bowel Disorders

Matching

1.	C ✓	6.	I ✓
2.	E ✓	7.	F ✓
3.	H ✓	8.	A ✓
4.	J ✓	9.	G ✓
5.	D ✓	10.	B ✓

Learning Outcomes

1. Diarrhea can result either from impaired water absorption or from increased water secretion into the bowel.

2. Dairy products, fruit juices, table sugar, coffee, and cola drinks can aggravate chronic diarrhea.

3. Older adults should be taught to increase dietary fiber to provide bulk, and drink six to eight glasses of water per day to assist in elimination. They should also remain as active as possible and not resist the urge to defecate when it is felt. The older adult should also be instructed when to contact their primary care physician regarding changes in their bowel habits.

4. Saline, tap-water, soap-suds, phosphate, and oil-retention are types of enemas.

5. Irritable bowel syndrome is a motility disorder characterized by alternating periods of constipation and diarrhea.

6. Before a small bowel series, the client may be restricted to a low-residue diet and receive a tap-water enema. The client will be instructed to avoid food, fluids, and smoking for at least eight hours before the exam. The client needs to know that the test requires several hours to complete, and that barium is instilled through a weighted tube inserted into the small bowel. Increase fluids after the test to expel the barium; stool will be chalky white for up to 72 hours after the exam due to the barium. The color will return to normal once the barium is excreted.

7. Malabsorption is ineffective intestinal absorption of nutrients. It usually occurs with disorders of the small intestine.

8. Manifestations of peritonitis include: diffuse or localized pain, tenderness with rebound, boardlike rigidity, diminished or absent bowel sounds, distention, nausea, fever, tachycardia, and restlessness.

9. Stool specimens, blood work, colonoscopies, and upper GI series with small bowel follow-through are some tests used to diagnose Crohn's disease.

10. Risk factors for colorectal cancer include: over 50 years old, family history, polyps of the rectum or colon, IBS, smoking, alcohol consumption, obesity, and high-fat, low-fiber diet.

Apply What You Learned

1. Nursing diagnoses for this client would include: Risk for Deficient Fluid Volume, Imbalanced Nutrition, Disturbed Body Image, and Diarrhea.
2. The information given is normal because the client is slowly advancing her diet to prevent further irritations, has no present complaints of loose stools or pain, and the abdomen is slightly distended, which indicates that the inflammation is resolving. Her blood pressure is not a factor because it is within normal limits.
3. Along with dietary modifications, the client should be instructed on stress reduction techniques and management. The client should be taught about the short- and long-term effects regarding the illness. Discuss the increased risk for colorectal cancer and the need for medical follow-up.

Multiple Choice

1.	C	6.	A	11.	C
2.	A	7.	D	12.	A
3.	B	8.	B	13.	B
4.	D	9.	C	14.	C
5.	C	10.	C	15.	B

Chapter 27 Caring for Clients With Gallbladder, Liver, and Pancreatic Disorders

Matching

1.	G	6.	J
2.	C	7.	F
3.	E	8.	B
4.	A	9.	H
5.	I	10.	D

Learning Outcomes

1. Age, family history, race, obesity, high cholesterol, female, and sickle cell anemia are risk factors for gallstones.
2. Biliary colic is a severe, steady pain in the right upper quadrant of the abdomen.
3. Some high-fat foods to avoid in cholelithiasis are: whole milk products, deep-fried foods, bacon, gravies, most nuts, chocolate, and snack foods such as potato chips.
4. Hepatitis is an inflammation of the liver. It is usually caused by a virus, but also may be caused by alcohol, toxins, or gallbladder disease. It can be acute or chronic in nature. Some types of hepatitis include: Hepatitis A, B, C, HDV, and E.

5. Jaundice occurs when serum bilirubin levels are high, which causes the skin, mucous membranes, and sclera of the eyes to appear yellow.
6. Health care workers, injection drug users, people on hemodialysis, recipients of clotting factors, and people at risk for sexual transmission should be vaccinated for Hepatitis B.
7. In cirrhosis, functional liver cells are destroyed, disrupting the metabolic functions of the liver. Lost cells are replaced by scar tissue that forms constrictive bands within liver lobules and disrupts blood flow within the liver. Impaired blood flow leads to portal hypertension and ultimately leads to liver failure.
8. Diagnostic testing for cirrhosis includes: CBC, liver function tests, blood chemistries, coagulation studies, ultrasound, liver biopsy, and an upper endoscopy.
9. In acute pancreatitis, the client presents with severe epigastric pain that may radiate to the back. The client may have nausea, vomiting, decreased bowel sounds, tachycardia, cool skin, elevated WBCs, and low magnesium. Chronic pancreatitis will present with elevated glucose levels, elevated amylase and lipase, constipation, anorexia, vomiting, weight loss, and persistent episodes of upper abdominal pain radiating to the back.
10. Lab tests for pancreatic disorders include: serum amylase, serum lipase, urine amylase, serum calcium, serum magnesium, white blood cells, and carcinoembryonic antigen.

Apply What You Learned

1. Nursing interventions for this client will include: daily weight before breakfast, dietician consult, assessment of mental status and report changes, measure abdominal girth every shift, bleeding precautions, keep head of bed elevated and legs elevated as tolerated, and utilize home health for follow-up.
2. The nurse needs to assess the ability and willingness of the wife to help with food preparation, follow-up medical care, and family responsibilities. Support groups such as Alcoholics Anonymous should be suggested. The wife should be made aware of social services and home health agencies that can offer assistance. The wife must also be aware of the discharge instructions set forth by the physician so that she may help her husband understand the treatment plan. The wife needs to understand the prognosis of the illness so as to provide the best care and quality of life to her husband.
3. Excess Fluid Volume, Imbalanced Nutrition, Disturbed Thought Processes, and Ineffective Protection are some nursing diagnoses related to this client.

Multiple Choice

1. A
2. A
3. D
4. B
5. D

6. C
7. A ✓
8. B
9. B
10. C

11. D ✓
12. A ✓
13. D
14. B ✓
15. A ✓

Chapter 28 The Urinary System and Assessment

Matching

1.	D	6.	I
2.	C	7.	G
3.	F	8.	J
4.	H	9.	A
5.	E	10.	B

Learning Outcomes

1. Nephrons are the functional units of the kidneys. Each kidney contains at least 1 million nephrons which process blood to make urine.
2. The ureters move urine from the kidney to the bladder by peristaltic waves. The ureters contain smooth muscle and are innervated by the autonomic nervous system. They are bilateral tubes that are about 10–12 inches long.
3. Glomerular filtration is a passive process in which fluid and solutes move from the blood in the glomerulus into Bowman's capsule. The amount of fluid filtered from the blood into the capsule per minute is called the glomerular filtration rate.
4. Normal GFR in adults is 120–125 mL/min.
5. Dysuria is painful urination. Nocturia is urinating more than once during the night, and hematuria is blood in the urine.
6. Lab tests used are: BUN, serum creatinine, creatinine clearance, and serum albumin.
7. Uroflowmetry is used to evaluate voiding and function of the lower urinary tract. It generally is used to evaluate retention and incontinence. It is non-invasive and measures the volume and rate of urine flow.
8. The 24-hour urine specimen is urine that is saved in a container for a 24-hour period. All urine must be collected or the test must be restarted. The specimen is kept in the refrigerator. The first urine collected is discarded. Notes should be placed in the client's bathroom, over the bed, on the chart and in the Kardex so that all persons know the test is in progress. Appropriate documentation regarding the specimen must be complete.
9. Inform the client and family that the procedure takes about 30–45 minutes and that local or general anesthesia may be used. The client may feel pressure or an urge to urinate as the scope is inserted. Burning on urination for a day or two after the procedure is considered normal. The client will need to notify the physician if the urine remains bloody, if there is bright red bleeding, if the client has a fever, or flank pain. Increasing the fluids will decrease pain and difficulty with urination and reduce the risk of infection.
10. Components involved in urine studies are: urinalysis, culture and sensitivity, 24-hour urine tests, electrolytes, protein, and creatinine.

Apply What You Learned

1. For a 24-hour urine test, verify the physician's order, obtain a specimen container with preservative (if indicated). Label with identifying data, the test, time started, and time of completion. Post notices on chart, Kardex, on the door, over the bed, over the toilet and alert all personnel that all urine is to be saved. At start time, have client empty bladder completely and discard urine. Save and refrigerate all urine for the next 24 hours. At the end of collection, have client empty the bladder one last time. Take entire specimen container with requisition to the lab. Chart appropriately. Remember that if one urine is missed, the test must be restarted.

2. A CT may be done to visualize structures of the urinary tract. A renal scan may be done to evaluate blood vessels and perfusion of the kidneys and ureters. Also, an ultrasound may be done to examine the size, shape, and position of the bladder and kidneys.

3. The physician is going to evaluate the status of sodium, chloride, potassium, calcium, and magnesium in the blood. Creatinine and protein will be evaluated also to help identify kidney disease.

Multiple Choice

1. C	6. C	11. B
2. C	7. A	12. C
3. B	8. B	13. D
4. D	9. C	14. A
5. C	10. A	15. A

Chapter 29 Caring for Clients With Renal and Urinary Tract Disorders

Matching

1. C	6. B
2. E	7. J
3. A	8. D
4. G	9. H
5. I	10. F

Learning Outcomes

1. Urinary incontinence is involuntary urination. It is common among older adults.

2. The types of incontinences are: Stress, urge, overflow, reflex, and functional incontinence.

3. Older adults with UTIs may be asymptomatic, or may present with nocturia, incontinence, confusion, behavior change, lethargy, anorexia, or "just not feeling right."

4. Azotemia is an increased blood level of nitrogenous waste including urea and creatinine.

5. Manifestations of urinary stones include: dull, aching flank pain, nausea, vomiting, cool, clammy skin, pain radiating to suprapubic region, groin, scrotum, or labia.

6. Goose, organ meats, sardines, herring, venison, chicken, crab, pork, salmon, and veal are all high in purines.

7. Impaired Urinary Elimination, Risk for Impaired Skin Integrity, and Disturbed Body Image are nursing diagnoses related to bladder cancer.

8. Dialysis is diffusion of solutes across a semipermeable membrane from an area of higher concentration to one of lower concentration. It compensates for the kidneys' inability to eliminate excess water and solutes.

9. Renal failure is a condition in which the kidneys are unable to remove accumulated waste products from the blood. It may be acute or chronic, and lead to fluid and electrolyte imbalance.

10. Maintain accurate I&O records, weigh the client daily, document vital signs at least every four hours, frequently assess heart and breath sounds, place in Fowler's position, restrict fluids as ordered, administer meds with meals, turn frequently, provide good skin care, administer diuretics as ordered, and monitor serum electrolytes as ordered.

Apply What You Learned

1. The nurse would explain that the kidneys are no longer able to remove waste products from the blood. If the cause is known, explain that to the client and family by using lay terms. The dialysis will be done to remove the waste products that the kidneys no longer can. The dialysis will act as the "filter."
To ensure understanding, ask the client for a return demonstration on information given and correct them when necessary. Keeping them informed will lead to a better outcome and improved cooperation.

2. The client's blood is pumped to a dialyzing unit where it moves past a semipermeable membrane. A solution, dialysate, is warmed to body temperature and passed along the other side of the membrane. Solutes diffuse through the membrane and into the dialysate. Excess water is removed from the blood by creating a higher fluid pressure on the blood side of the membrane.

3. Excess Fluid Volume, Imbalanced Nutrition, Risk for Infection, and Disturbed Body Image are nursing diagnoses that pertain to this client.

Multiple Choice

1. C	6. C	11. A
2. C	7. D	12. C
3. B	8. D	13. A
4. A	9. A	14. C
5. C	10. A	15. B

Chapter 30 The Reproductive System and Assessment

Matching

1. A
2. D
3. E
4. G
5. F

6. B
7. I
8. J
9. H
10. C

Learning Outcomes

1. The reproductive system in men includes the paired testes, the scrotum, ducts, glans, and penis.
2. The internal organs of the female reproductive system include the ovaries, fallopian tubes, uterus, and vagina.
3. Estrogens are steroid hormones essential to the development and maintenance of secondary sex characteristics.
4. Mammography is used to screen for breast cancer in women who have no symptoms. It can detect tumors that are too small to be detected by a clinical breast exam or breast self-exam.
5. Pelvic ultrasound is used to identify tumors and to monitor ovulation in women. Abdominal and vaginal approaches are used. For the vaginal approach, the transducer is covered with a condom and coated with transducer gel.
6. This test is used on men to assess the prostate gland, urethra, seminal vesicles, and vas deferens. It may also be used to guide a needle biopsy of the prostate. It is sometimes performed under sedation.
7. The prostate gland is the size of a walnut and encircles the urethra just below the urinary bladder. Secretions of the prostate gland make up about one-third of the volume in semen.
8. The ovarian cycle has three phases. The follicular phase lasts from the 1st to the 10th day of the cycle. The ovulatory phase lasts from the 11th to the 14th day, ending with ovulation, and the luteal phase lasts from the 14th to the 28th day.
9. Spermatogenesis is sperm production. It begins with puberty and continues throughout a man's life, with several hundred million sperm produced daily. Spermatogenesis takes 64 to 72 days.
10. Seminal fluid is made of secretions from the seminal vesicles, the epididymis, prostate gland, and Cowper's gland. It nourishes the sperm, provides bulk, and increases its alkalinity.

Apply What You Learned

1. The menstrual cycle, or ovarian cycle, has three phases and lasts 28 days. Days 1–10 are the follicular phase that involve the primary, secondary, and vasicular follicles. Ovulation occurs in the next phase and lasts from the 11th to the 14th day. This is the time when a woman is the most fertile. The luteal phase lasts from the 14th day to the 28th day, sets up the corpus luteum, and degenerates the corpus luteum. This is when the period occurs.

2. The first thing the nurse needs to do is provide as much privacy as possible. Then initiate friendly dialogue so that trust can be achieved. Then the nurse can ask the teen what she knows and believes to be true about menstruation. The interview process may take place with or without a parent/guardian present. The physical exam is usually accompanied by the parent.

Multiple Choice

1.	C ✓	6.	D	11.	D ✓
2.	D	7.	C ✓	12.	A ✓
3.	B ✓	8.	A ✓	13.	B
4.	A ✓	9.	B	14.	C
5.	C	10.	D ✓	15.	A ✓

Chapter 31 Caring for Male Clients With Reproductive System Disorders

Matching

1.	D	6.	J
2.	G	7.	H
3.	E	8.	B
4.	C	9.	F
5.	I	10.	A

Learning Outcomes

1. Benign prostatic hyperplasia is the enlargement of the prostate gland and affects most men over the age of 50. The incidence of BPH increases with age.
2. Manifestations of prostate cancer include: reduced urinary stream, increased frequency, erectile dysfunction, bone or joint pain, back pain, lower extremity weakness, weight loss, fatigue, anemia, and bowel or bladder dysfunction.
3. Digital Rectal Exam, DRE, is a screening tool to identify an enlarged prostate. The lab will run serum PSA levels and possibly test a tissue sample. The physician may also order imaging studies such as a CT or MRI to identify possible tumors.
4. Orchiectomy is a removal of the testes.
5. With retropubic prostatectomy, the prostate gland is removed through an abdominal incision and the bladder is left intact. In a suprapubic prostatectomy, the prostate gland is removed through an abdominal incision into the bladder. With a perineal prostatectomy, the prostate gland is removed through a perineal incision between the scrotum and anus.
6. Impaired Urinary Elimination, Risk for Incontinence, Sexual Dysfunction, and Pain are nursing diagnoses for prostate dysfunction.
7. Testicular torsion is a twisting of the tests and spermatic cord, and is a potential medical emergency. Boys and young men up to age 20 are at greatest risk for testicular torsion; the cause is unclear.
8. Cryptorchidism is failure of one or both testes to descend through the inguinal ring into the scrotum.

9. Testicular cancer is the most common cancer in men between the ages of 15 and 35. It is one of the most treatable, with a cure rate of greater than 90%. The cause is unknown, but risk factors can include a family history, undescended testicles, race, and ethnicity. Beginning at age 15, all men should perform monthly testicular self-exams to assess for lumps or irregularities. Testicular cancer grows within the testicle and eventually replaces most of the normal tissue. Usually only one testicle is affected.

10. Erectile dysfunction or impotence, is the inability to attain and maintain an erection that allows satisfactory sexual intercourse.

Apply What You Learned

1. This client will have labs done to evaluate the PSA level. The physician may also order a CT or MRI to evaluate the nodule for size, shape, and location. A urinalysis will also be ordered to rule out infection and calculi.

2. This client is a candidate for a retropubic prostatectomy. In this procedure, the prostate gland will be removed through an abdominal incision and the bladder will be left intact. The client will have an indwelling catheter post-procedure to allow appropriate healing.

3. The nurse will talk to the client about possible stress incontinence after the catheter is removed. Post-operative complications such as infection will need to be discussed so that the client and his wife know when to notify the physician. The nurse needs to reinforce follow-up care to monitor the disease and the healing process.

Multiple Choice

1.	D	6.	C	11.	B
2.	B	7.	A	12.	B
3.	A	8.	A	13.	C
4.	B	9.	B	14.	A
5.	A	10.	D	15.	D

Chapter 32 Caring for Female Clients With Reproductive System Disorders

Matching

1.	B	6.	H
2.	D	7.	J
3.	F	8.	I
4.	A	9.	G
5.	E	10.	C

Learning Outcomes

1. Menopause is the period during which menstruation permanently ceases. It marks the natural end of reproduction.

2. HRT is often used to relieve unpleasant manifestations of menopause and reduce some of the risks associated with estrogen deficiency. HRT relieves hot flashes and night sweats, and decreases vaginal dryness. Perineal tissue atrophy, which can lead to painful intercourse and urinary incontinence, can also be relieved with HRT.

3. PMS is a symptom complex of irritability, depression, edema, and breast tenderness preceding menses. Risk factors for PMS include major life stressors, being over 30 and depression. The actual cause is unknown but it is thought to involve imbalances of estrogen and progesterone.

4. A hysterectomy is a removal of the uterus. The ovaries are usually left in place unless other conditions warrant their removal.

5. Endometriosis is a common condition in which endometrial tissue is found outside the uterus. Endometrial tissue may be found on the ovary and other pelvic organs or tissues, and rarely in other organs such as the lungs. The cause is unknown, but it may be caused by backflow of menstrual blood carrying endometrial cells through the fallopian tubes into the pelvis.

6. Diagnostic testing used regarding ovarian cysts include: LH, FSH and serum testosterone, glucose tolerance tests, and a laparoscopy.

7. Vaginitis is an inflammation or infection of the vagina. Such infections are common and may be fungal, protozoal, or bacterial.

8. PID is an infection of the pelvic organs. It is usually caused by infection with *Neisseria gonorrhoeae* and/or *Chlamydia trachomatis*. Clients with PID are often infected with more than one organism. It is a major cause of infertility. It usually affects young, sexually active women who have multiple partners.

9. Cervical cancer is common. Early detection and intervention have substantially reduced the incidence of invasive cervical cancer as well as the number of deaths due to cervical cancer. Most occurrences are related to infection of the cervix with human papillomavirus (HPV). Other risk factors for cervical cancer include early sexual experience, multiple sex partners, HIV infection, unprotected sex, smoking, and a poor diet. Early cancer causes no symptoms. With progression, the woman may notice pain in the back or thighs, hematuria, bloody stools, anemia, and weight loss.

10. A uterine prolapse is caused by stretching of the ligaments that normally support the uterus within the pelvis. Increased pressure within the abdomen also can lead to uterine prolapse.

Apply What You Learned

1. This client's risk factors are nipple discharge, breast pain, skin rash, and family history.

2. Mammograms, ultrasounds, CT, MRI, cytologic exams, and tissue biopsy are diagnostic tests done to confirm breast cancer.

3. Nursing diagnoses include: Decisional Conflict regarding treatment options, Grieving, Risk for Infection, Risk for Injury, and Risk for Disturbed Body Image.

4. During the grieving process, the nurse must listen attentively to expressions of loss and observe for nonverbal cues. The nurse must also spend time with the client and not rush interactions. The nurse needs to explain that periods

of depression, anger, and denial are normal and expected. The nurse needs to locate community resources and ensure that the client has support from family.

Multiple Choice

1.	D	6.	A	11.	B
2.	B	7.	C	12.	C
3.	D	8.	A	13.	A
4.	A	9.	D	14.	B
5.	B	10.	C	15.	B

Chapter 33 Caring for Clients With Sexually Transmitted Infections

Matching

1.	G	6.	I
2.	E	7.	B
3.	H	8.	A
4.	F	9.	C
5.	J	10.	D

Learning Outcomes

1. Any infection transmitted by sexual contact—including vaginal, oral, and anal intercourse—is known as a sexually transmitted infection (STI) or disease (STD).
2. Risk factors for STIs include: personal history or partner history of STI, teen sexual activity, use of oral contraceptives, unprotected sex, multiple sex partners, and pregnancy.
3. Chlamydial infections are thought to be the most common STI and the leading cause of pelvic inflammatory disease. It is a bacterium that behaves like a virus, reproducing only within the host cell. It is spread by any sexual contact. It is asymptomatic in most women until it has invaded the uterus and uterine tubes. Men are also asymptomatic and eventually can present with urethral discharge.
4. Females with gonorrhea are often asymptomatic, but may have vaginal discharge, abnormal menses, and dysuria. Men may have dysuria, increased urinary frequency, and purulent urethral discharge.
5. Some nursing diagnoses related to STIs include: Ineffective Health Maintenance, Impaired Skin Integrity, Risk for Injury, Anxiety, Situational Low Self-Esteem, Sexual Dysfunction, and Impaired Social Interaction.
6. The best preventative measure against STIs is abstinence. However, when there is concern about preventing STIs, it's important to know that the more sexual partners you have, the greater the risk of contracting an STI.

Use condoms, vaginal spermicides, and lubricants with each sexual encounter. Seek out a physician if you suspect an STI, and go back for follow-up care. Do not have sex until you and your partners are completely cleared to do so by a physician.

7. Genital herpes is a chronic and often asymptomatic STI. Currently, no cure is available for genital herpes. It is spread by vaginal, anal, or oral-genital contact. It has an incubation period of three to seven days. Within a week of exposure, painful red papules appear in the genital area.

8. Syphilis, if not treated, can lead to blindness, paralysis, mental illness, cardio-vascular damage, and death. Penicillin has significantly reduced the incidence of syphilis. Syphilis often occurs with one or more other STIs, such as HIV or chlamydia. It begins with an ulcer at this site which may become a rash, especially on the palms of the hands or soles of the feet. Mucous patches may appear in the oral cavity along with a sore throat. Flu-like symptoms may also be present. The latent stage of syphilis can last up to 50 years. During this stage, no symptoms are apparent and it is not transmissible by sexual contact. It can be transmitted through blood, however.

9. Females may be asymptomatic or may have frothy, excessive vaginal discharge, erythema, edema, and pruritus. Males usually are asymptomatic also, though they may have urethritis, penile lesions, or inflammation.

10. Reportable STIs include: syphilis, gonorrhea, and AIDS. Chlamydia is reportable in most but not all states.

Apply What You Learned

1. The student nurse can create an environment in which the client feels respected and safe to discuss concerns about the disease and its effect on the client's life. Providing privacy and confidentiality along with compassionate communication are key with this age group. The student nurse must also be nonjudgmental and supportive while informing the teens that an STI is not a punishment but a consequence of sexual behavior.

2. Syphilis, gonorrhea, and AIDS are STIs that need to be reported.

3. The student nurse will inform the teens that risk factors for STIs include: pregnancy, multiple sexual partners, unprotected sexual activity, and a history of STI.

Multiple Choice

1.	A	6.	A	11.	D
2.	B	7.	D	12.	D
3.	D	8.	A	13.	D
4.	D	9.	B	14.	A
5.	D	10.	D	15.	B

Matching

1.	B	6.	A
2.	B	7.	C
3.	C	8.	C
4.	B	9.	D
5.	B	10.	A

Learning Outcomes

1. The primary function of the endocrine system is to regulate the body's internal environment. This regulation is maintained through the function of various hormones within the endocrine system. The hormones regulate growth, reproduction, metabolism, and fluid/electrolyte balance.
2. TSH, T3, T4, growth hormone, serum Ca, phosphorus, HgbA1C, and blood glucose, as well as urine tests for glucose and ketones, will be performed.
3. An MRI uses a magnet and radio frequency signals to elicit a response from hydrogen nuclei. As a result, tumors of the pituitary gland and hypothalamus can be identified.
4. The thyroid gland increases metabolic rates and lowers serum calcium levels. It is shaped like a butterfly and sits on either side of the trachea.
5. The hypothalmus controls the anterior pituitary function by regulating temperature, fluid volume, and growth. It also responds to pain, pleasure, hunger, and thirst stimuli.
6. The pancreas is the primary organ involved in diabetes. It is located behind the stomach between the spleen and duodenum. It serves two major functions. Acini cells secrete digestive enzymes into the duodenum, and the islets of Langerhans release insulin and glucagon into the bloodstream.
7. Insulin's primary function is to regulate blood glucose levels. Insulin release increases when blood glucose levels rise and decreases when blood glucose levels fall. When a person eats food, insulin levels rise in minutes, peak in 30–60 minutes, and return to baseline in 2–3 hours.
8. Exophthalmos is forward protrusion of the eyeballs. It is diagnosed upon physical examination for some endocrine disorders.
9. The client must fast during the test and drink 75 grams of glucose. This test determines the level of glucose 2 hours after drinking the 75 grams. Levels should return to normal, but a level higher than 200 mg/dL indicates diabetes.
10. The adrenal cortex stimulates gluconeogenesis and increases blood glucose levels. It also regulates blood volume and electrolytes.

Apply What You Learned

1. Graves' Disease is an autoimmune disorder, which is the most common cause of hyperthyroidism. It develops 10 times more often in women under the age of 40 than in the general population.
2. Graves' is due to hyperthyroidism, so there may be associated hand tremors, nervousness, and insomnia. The client may also experience blurry vision, tachycardia, fine hair, weight loss, and muscle weakness.
3. Treatment for Graves' includes antithyroid medications, iodine sources, and beta-adrenergic blockers.

Multiple Choice

1.	D	6.	F	11.	A
2.	E	7.	H	12.	D
3.	B	8.	C	13.	C
4.	G	9.	J	14.	A
5.	A	10.	I	15.	B

Chapter 35 Caring for Clients With Endocrine Disorders

Matching

1.	D	6.	F
2.	E	7.	A
3.	B	8.	C
4.	G	9.	J
5.	H	10.	I

Learning Outcomes

1. Diabetes insipidus is a condition that results from antidiuretic hormone insufficiency. There are two types: neurogenic and nephrogenic. The client will present with extreme thirst, polyuria, weakness, and dehydration.
2. Also called a thyroid storm, thyrotoxic crisis is an extreme state of hyperthyroidism that is rare today. This disorder may result from untreated hyperthyroid, infection, diabetic ketoacidosis, physical/emotional trauma, or thyroid surgery. It is life-threatening and requires immediate medical attention.
3. A goiter is an enlargement due to iodine deficiency, most commonly seen on the neck.
4. The client with myxedema coma will present with seizures, lethargy which quickly progresses to a coma, and hypothermia. This is a life-threatening emergency.
5. Tetany is a continuous spasm of muscles.
6. Cushing's syndrome is a chronic disorder in which the adrenal cortex produces excessive amounts of the hormone cortisol. It is more common in women between the ages of 20 and 50.

7. The client with Addison's will present with bronzing over the knuckles, knees, and elbows. Muscle weakness, irregular pulse, lethargy, depression, anorexia, and salt cravings may also be present.
8. Nursing diagnoses for endocrine disorders could include: Disturbed Thought Processes, Hypothermia, Constipation, Activity Intolerance, and Risk for Impaired Skin Integrity.
9. Pheochromocytoma is a benign tumor of the adrenal medulla. The tumor produces excessive amounts of epinephrine and stimulates the sympathetic nervous system.
10. Corticosteroids are the main medication class for the treatment of Addison's disease. Examples would be: prednisone, Solu-Medrol, and Decadron.

Apply What You Learned

1. Tests for this client would include T3, T4, TSH levels along with a routine CBC and CMP.
2. The diagnosis of hypothyroidism would be made due to the manifestations of weight gain, loss of appetite, and always being cold.
3. Levothyroxine is one of the most common medications used in the treatment of hypothyroidism. Client education regarding body changes, dietary modifications, and rest periods will be part of the treatment plan.

Multiple Choice

1. B	6. B	11. A
2. C	7. B	12. B
3. B	8. A	13. A
4. A	9. C	14. C
5. C	10. B	15. A

Chapter 36 Caring for Clients With Diabetes Mellitus

Matching

1. F	6. G
2. H	7. D
3. E	8. B
4. I	9. C
5. J	10. A

Learning Outcomes

1. Type 1 diabetes is a state of absolute insulin deficiency. It usually occurs before childhood, and the client is prone to developing ketoacidosis. These clients are insulin dependent. Type 2 is a state of sufficient insulin to prevent ketoacidosis but insufficient to lower blood glucose levels. It usually occurs

after the age of 30, and most clients are obese. They are not insulin dependent but may require insulin.

2. Polyuria, polydipsia, polyphagia, weight loss, fatigue, and malaise are some manifestations of type 1 diabetes.

3. Glycosuria is excess glucose in the urine.

4. The four types of insulin are: rapid-acting, short-acting, intermediate-acting, and long-acting.

5. Long-acting insulin, such as Ultralente, has an onset of 4–6 hours with a peak time of 18–24 hours. The duration of this medication is 36 hours.

6. When administering insulin, be sure to discard any vial whose expiration date has passed. Be sure to check the client's blood glucose 30 minutes before giving insulin and check type and dose with another nurse. Keep a record of blood glucose levels and monitor for signs and symptoms of hyper/hypoglycemia.

7. The client should be instructed to maintain caloric intake to coincide with their body weight. Artificial sweeteners such as Sweet & Low and Nutrasweet should be used instead of pure sugar. Diabetics should be taught to have 15–20% of their daily intake in protein and have 20–35 grams of fiber daily. They should be taught to limit alcohol and have less than 10% of their daily calories from saturated fats.

8. Ketonuria is a presence of ketones in the urine, which usually occurs when the blood glucose is greater than 250 mg/dL.

9. When a client is in a hyperosmolar hyperglycemic state, they will present with severely elevated blood glucose levels, extreme dehydration, and an altered level of consciousness.

10. Peripheral vascular disease may present with loss of hair on lower legs, shininess of the skin, cold feet, thick toenails, diminished pulses, pain at rest, and intermittent claudication.

Apply What You Learned

1. The nurse should request a dietary consult with a diabetes education specialist. The nurse should also provide examples of sugar substitutes, proteins, and fiber-rich foods. The client should be taught to order out in moderation, and to add fruits and vegetables as snacks. The nurse should instruct the client on staying well hydrated by drinking water, especially when the client wants a sugary snack. Ensure that the dietician can provide real-world examples of lunches that will suit his lifestyle.

2. This client will receive insulin by injection to cover the 312 blood glucose reading. Monitoring and documentation should be completed regarding the urine output and other signs and symptoms of hyperglycemia. The nurse should monitor for signs of altered levels of consciousness and visual disturbances. A re-check of the blood glucose should be done according to facility policy or as the physician requests.

3. The client needs to be educated on the importance of keeping the feet clean and dry, especially in between the toes. The feet should be inspected daily for cracks in the skin. The nurse should instruct the client to never go barefoot, and to always wear appropriately fitting shoes and white cotton socks.

The client should be taught to cut toenails after washing because they will be soft, and to cut them straight across to avoid ingrown toenails. The physician will inspect the feet upon each follow-up visit, so let the client know that he will be asked to remove his socks and shoes.

Multiple Choice

1. A	6. B	11. A
2. B	7. D	12. A
3. C	8. D	13. C
4. A	9. A	14. C
5. A	10. C	15. A

Chapter 37 The Nervous System and Assessment

Matching

1. E	6. J
2. D	7. H
3. B	8. I
4. C	9. A
5. G	10. F

Learning Outcomes

1. Myelin sheath is a white fatty substance that protects and insulates axons.
2. The three layers of meninges are: dura mater, arachnoid, and pia mater.
3. The cerebellum is connected to the midbrain, pons, and medulla. Like the cerebrum, it has two hemispheres. It coordinates involuntary muscle activity and fine motor movements, as well as balance and posture.
4. A reflex is an involuntary motor response to a stimulus.
5. The ANS is part of the peripheral nervous system. It is responsible for maintaining the body's internal homeostasis. It regulates respiration, heart rate, digestion, urinary excretion, body temperature, and sexual function.
6. Cheyne–Stokes respirations are periods of apnea for 10–60 seconds, followed by a gradual increase in rate and depth of breathing.
7. Age-related changes in vision include decreased corneal sensation and tear secretion, constriction of the pupil, decreased elasticity and increased density of the lens, loss of rods at periphery of retina, and loss of fat and subcutaneous tissue around the eyes.
8. Dysphagia is difficulty swallowing.
9. The tenth cranial nerve is the vagus nerve. It is responsible for the function of swallowing, controls heart and respiratory rates and digestion, and controls the sensation in pharynx and larynx.
10. A neurotransmitter is a chemical that either helps the impulse cross the synapse or stops it.

Apply What You Learned

1. Cranial nerves nine and ten are involved with swallowing.
2. The cranial nerves related to eyeball movement are three, four, and six.

Multiple Choice

1.	D	6.	C	11.	D
2.	A	7.	D	12.	A
3.	B	8.	B	13.	A
4.	C	9.	B	14.	B
5.	A	10.	C	15.	B

Chapter 38 Caring for Clients With Intracranial Disorders

Matching

1.	H	6.	C
2.	J	7.	A
3.	I	8.	G
4.	B	9.	D
5.	E	10.	F

Learning Outcomes

1. A hematoma is an accumulation of blood.
2. Manifestations of concussion include immediate loss of consciousness for less than five minutes, drowsiness, confusion, dizziness, headache, and blurred or double vision.
3. The three types of hematomas are epidural, subdural, and intracerebral.
4. Someone with an altered level of consciousness may be disoriented to person, place, and time. The person may have a short attention span and poor memory, or may appear restless, agitated, and combative.
5. Brain tumors are abnormal growths within the cranium. Their cause is unknown, but prolonged exposure to certain chemicals and radiation increases the incidence.
6. Manifestations related to brain tumors include personality changes, inappropriate behavior, impaired judgment, recent memory loss, motor deficits, expressive aphasia, seizures, headache, and visual deficits.
7. A CVA is also called a brain attack or stroke. It leads to neurologic deficits from decreased blood supply to a local area of the brain.
8. A seizure is a brief disruption of brain function caused by abnormal electrical activity in the nerve cells of the brain. They may occur as an isolated event or as part of a disorder.
9. Status epilepticus is a continuous period of tonic–clonic seizures in which the client does not regain consciousness. It is considered a life-threatening emergency that could result in permanent brain damage.

10. Meningitis is an inflammation of the meninges of the brain and spinal cord. Once bacteria or virus enters the CNS, it begins an inflammatory response in the meninges, CSF, and ventricles. Recovery is usually uneventful.

Apply What You Learned

1. The likely diagnosis for this client is CVA.
2. Diagnostic tests that the nurse would expect to see ordered include: CT scan, MRI, cerebral arteriography, Doppler ultrasound, PET, and lumbar puncture.
3. The treatment plan for this client will include antiplatelet medications such as Plavix. Low-dose aspirin taken daily may also be utilized. If there are residual effects from the CVA, the client may require physical, occupational, or speech therapies. They may need to perform the therapy in a long-term care facility or rehabilitation center.

Multiple Choice

1.	B	6.	C	11.	A
2.	B	7.	A	12.	D
3.	D	8.	B	13.	C
4.	C	9.	D	14.	B
5.	D	10.	B	15.	C

Chapter 39 Caring for Clients With Degenerative Neurologic and Spinal Cord Disorders

Matching

1.	D	6.	G	
2.	J	7.	A	
3.	E	8.	B	
4.	I	9.	F	
5.	H	10.	C	

Learning Outcomes

1. Alzheimer's disease is a progressive, irreversible deterioration of the brain. It is characterized by a gradual loss of intellectual functioning. It is the most common type of dementia.
2. Sundowning syndrome is behavior characterized by increased agitation, disorientation to time, and wandering during afternoon and evening hours.
3. The purpose of plasmapheresis is to remove T lymphocytes that cause inflammation.
4. Manifestations related to Parkinson's include: tremors, rigidity of the neck, shoulders and trunk, bradykinesia, drooling, excess sweating on face and neck, oily skin, memory loss, and inability to initiate voluntary movements.

5. Huntington's disease is a progressive, inherited neurologic disease. There is no cure, and each child who has a parent with HD has a 50% chance of inheriting the disease. It involves a lack of a neurotransmitter, GABA, and eventually leads to personality changes, intellectual changes, and movement dysfunction.

6. ALS, Lou Gehrig's disease, involves loss of motor neurons in the spinal cord and brainstem. When these impulses cannot be sent to the brain, they lose strength and atrophy. Although body function decreases, the person remains mentally alert.

7. Rabies is a viral infection of the CNS caused by an animal bite.

8. Spinal cord injuries are usually due to trauma. The spinal cord provides a two-way path to conduct impulses between the brain and body. Spinal cord injury mechanisms include: hyperflexion, hyperextension, and cord compression. Most injuries occur in the lumbar and cervical regions, where the vertebrae are not protected by other parts of the skeleton, such as the rib cage or pelvis.

9. Autonomic dysreflexia is an exaggerated sympathetic response in clients with SCIs at or above the T6 level. The client develops a pounding headache, goosebumps, and anxiety.

10. Spinal cord tumors may be primary or secondary, benign, or malignant. Most of them occur in the thoracic and cervical areas. They compress the cord, spinal nerve roots, and surrounding blood vessels. Pain is often the first sign and is described as localized or radiating.

Apply What You Learned

1. Discuss the following topics with the client and family: avoiding stress, extreme heat or cold, and physical overexertion; medications and side effects; bowel and bladder schedule; ways to prevent complications such as pressure ulcers; ways to cope with pain; importance of follow-up care; and community agencies that are availabe as the disease progresses.

2. The student nurse should encourage the client and family to express their feelings. Seek out a counselor if needed. Refer them to a support group and provide information about the National MS Society. Also refer them to state vocational rehabilitation agencies as needed.

Multiple Choice

1. A	6. B	11. C	
2. B	7. B	12. D	
3. D	8. B	13. D	
4. B	9. C	14. A	
5. A	10. A	15. D	

Matching

1.	A	6.	J
2.	H	7.	F
3.	I	8.	D
4.	E	9.	C
5.	B	10.	G

Learning Outcomes

1. Conjunctivitis is an inflammation of the conjunctiva and is a common eye disease.
2. Cataracts are the clouding of the lens of the eye that impairs vision. They are common, and most people over 65 have some cataracts. It usually affects both eyes, but each eye tends to develop at a different rate. As a cataract matures, both near and distance vision are affected. Details become obscured and light rays become scattered, causing a problem with glare and adjusting between light and dark environments.
3. Manifestations of glaucoma include: gradual loss of peripheral vision, blurred vision, halos around lights, difficulty focusing on near objects, possible nausea and vomiting, cornea clouded, and fixed pupils.
4. Face the client, so that the two of you are seated about two feet apart. Instruct the client to cover the right eye and focus on your face. Cover your left eye and focus on the client's face. Midway between the client and yourself, bring a light-colored object into the field of vision from the side. Ask the client to indicate when the object is seen. Check all visual fields of both eyes in this manner.
5. A detached retina is separation of the retina from the choroid, the vascular layer of the eye.
6. Macular degeneration is a common cause of blindness in older adults. With aging, the neurons of the macula may atrophy or separate from the choroid. When the macula is damaged, central vision becomes blurred and distorted, but peripheral vision remains intact. It usually affects activities such as reading and sewing.
7. To prevent external otitis: stay out of the water for 7–10 days or until completely healed, use earplugs to keep cold water out of ears, use a hair dryer on the lowest setting to dry ear canals after swimming, and do not insert cotton swabs or any other object into the ear canals.
8. Tinnitus is ringing in the ears.
9. Vertigo is a sensation of whirling or movement when there is none, and is the key symptom of inner ear disorders.
10. Disturbed Sensory Perception, Impaired Verbal Communication, and Social Isolation are nursing diagnoses related to hearing loss.

Apply What You Learned

1. The nurse needs to orient the client to his environment verbally and physically. Describe items within the area such as chairs, steps, and carpeting. Give the client verbal cues when they are performing a task so that they feel empowered to continue. Keep hallways and rooms free of clutter when the client is ambulating.
2. The family can orient the client as to the position of the food on the plate. Using the face of a clock is familiar to use as a reference. For example, carrots are at 3 o'clock. Juice is at twelve. This way, the client maintains independence and nutrition.
3. There are state, local, and national agencies to help coordinate services for the blind.

Multiple Choice

1. C	6. D	11. B
2. B	7. D	12. B
3. C	8. B	13. A
4. A	9. C	14. A
5. A	10. C	15. D

Chapter 41 The Musculoskeletal System and Assessment

Matching

1. F	6. H
2. E	7. A
3. J	8. D
4. I	9. G
5. B	10. C

Learning Outcomes

1. Ligaments are bands of connective tissue that connect bones to bones.
2. Three types of muscle tissue are: skeletal, smooth, and cardiac.
3. Adduction is to move toward the midline of the body while abduction is to move away from the midline of the body.
4. Ballottement is applying downward pressure with one hand placed just above the knee. With the other hand, tap the patella. Fluid in the knee causes the patella to rebound against the fingers.
5. ESR is the erythrocyte sedimentation rate, which is a nonspecific measure of inflammation.
6. Testing for calcium is important for monitoring the skeletal system because most of the body's calcium is in the bones and teeth. Adequate total body calcium is vital to maintain bone mass. Blood levels increase when calcium is released from the bone.

7. It is a test used to diagnose osteoporosis by measuring bone mineral density. They use special x-ray imaging techniques that expose the client to very low amounts of radiation and help predict fracture risk by comparing the individual's bone mass to that of a healthy 25–35-year-old person.

8. Arthroscopy uses a flexible fiberoptic endoscope to view joint structures and tissues. It is used to identify torn tendons or ligaments, an injured meniscus, inflammatory joint changes, and damaged cartilage.

9. Arthrocentesis is the procedure used to obtain fluid from a joint.

10. Normal phosphate levels are 2.5–4.5 mg/dL. It has an inverse relationship with calcium. When calcium levels are up, phosphate will be down, and vice versa.

Apply What You Learned

1. X-rays, lab tests to include ESR, CRP, Ca, Ph, U\uric acid, and RF, and perhaps arthrocentesis if fluid is present.

2. Yes, this client would be an appropriate candidate for arthroscopic surgery. This appears to be an inflammatory joint change and the procedure is used to identify such changes.

Multiple Choice

1.	B	6.	C	11.	B
2.	A	7.	B	12.	A
3.	C	8.	C	13.	B
4.	B	9.	B	14.	C
5.	A	10.	A	15.	A

Chapter 42 Caring for Clients With Musculoskeletal Trauma

Matching

1.	J	6.	H
2.	C	7.	F
3.	G	8.	B
4.	I	9.	E
5.	A	10.	D

Learning Outcomes

1. Characteristics of a sprain include: ligament injury, joint instability, pain, swelling, discoloration, and increased pain with joint use.

2. A fracture is a break in the continuity of a bone.

3. Compartment syndrome occurs when excess pressure restricts blood vessels and nerves within a compartment. It may be caused by bleeding or edema within the compartment or by external compression of the limb by a too-tight cast.

4. Carpal tunnel syndrome is one of the most common work-related injuries. It develops when the tunnel narrows, compressing and irritating the median nerve. This usually results from inflammation and swelling of structures in the wrist joint.

5. Phantom pain is felt along nerves of the body part that has been amputated. The exact cause is unknown, but it may be caused by trauma to the nerves serving the amputated part. The missing extremity feels numb, crushed, trapped, twisted, or burning. Management is challenging and often requires referral to a pain clinic.

6. To decrease fractures in older adults, monitor responses to medications, introduce assistive devices in stages as reflexes slow and gait alterations appear, address safety issues such as risks for falling, assess the need for in-home assistance, and make appropriate referrals to visiting nurses and home health aides.

7. Traction is use of a straightening or pulling force to return or maintain the fractured bones in normal position.

8. Manifestations of compartment syndrome include: pain, pallor, paresthesias, paresis, and pulselessness.

9. Fat emboli occur when fat globules lodge in a pulmonary vessel or the peripheral circulation. In the bloodstream, fat globules combine with platelets and travel to the brain, lungs, kidneys, and other organs, blocking small vessels and causing tissue ischemia.

10. RICE is an acronym that stands for: Rest, Ice, Compression, and Elevation.

Apply What You Learned

1. Encourage verbalization and validation of feelings. Contact the physician for a referral to a psychologist or social worker. Teach the importance of moving and ROM exercises to prevent contractures. Also encourage turning and lying in the prone position.

2. The nurse can contact social services who will assist the client with home health nurses and financial resources. The nurse should also contact the dietician to ensure the client is getting what he needs to promote wound healing.

Multiple Choice

1.	C	6.	B	11.	C
2.	D	7.	B	12.	A
3.	B	8.	A	13.	A
4.	C	9.	B	14.	B
5.	A	10.	C	15.	C

Matching

1.	E	6.	I
2.	F	7.	B
3.	G	8.	C
4.	H	9.	A
5.	D	10.	J

Learning Outcomes

1. A pathological fracture is a spontaneous fracture that occurs with little or no trauma.
2. Risks for osteomyelitis include: open fractures, puncture wounds, orthopedic surgery, soft tissue infection, pressure ulcers, impaired immune function, and diabetes.
3. Osteoarthritis is a degenerative joint disease characterized by progressive loss of joint cartilage in synovial joints. It is the most common type of arthritis and is a leading cause of disability in older adults.
4. Rheumatoid arthritis is a chronic, systemic inflammatory disorder that primarily affects the joints. It is a connective tissue disorder that affects more women than men and usually develops between the ages of 30 and 50.
5. Lupus erythematosus is a chronic inflammatory connective tissue disease. It affects multiple body systems and can range in severity from mild and episodic to a rapidly fatal disease. A cardinal sign of lupus is the butterfly rash on the face.
6. Fibromyalgia is a common rheumatic syndrome of musculoskeletal pain, stiffness, and tenderness.
7. MD is a group of inherited muscular diseases that cause progressive muscle degeneration and wasting. The most common form is Duchenne's, which is inherited from a recessive gene and transmitted from the mother to the male children. Muscle fiber atrophy, necrosis, regeneration, and fibrosis lead to progressive weakness of voluntary muscles in MD. As the disease progresses, the person develops difficulty ambulating and eventually becomes wheelchair-bound and finally bed-bound.
8. Multisystem effects of lupus include: butterfly rash on face, alopecia, depression, renal failure, photophobia, anemia, arthralgias, anorexia, pleurisy, dementia, and vasculitis.
9. Manifestations of rheumatoid arthritis include swelling, warmth, tenderness, and pain in the joints; limited range of motion and morning stiffness that lasts more than one hour; joint destruction; and deformity including nodules over the elbows, joints, and toes.
10. Arthralgia is localized joint pain and is the most common symptom of OA.

Apply What You Learned

1. Discharge teaching for this client would be to provide them with a list, including pictures, of the exercises and ROM the client is permitted to do. Referrals to home health and physical therapy along with a follow-up appointment with the surgeon should be scheduled in a timely manner to decrease complications. The client should be taught about pain control and when to call the physician.
2. Ask the client and his wife to recall the information that was reviewed with them. Ask them to demonstrate the exercises as well as what information they need when they call the physician.

Multiple Choice

1.	A	6.	C	11.	A
2.	D	7.	D	12.	C
3.	C	8.	D	13.	A
4.	A	9.	B	14.	B
5.	C	10.	D	15.	D

Chapter 44 The Integumentary System and Assessment

Matching

1.	E	6.	G
2.	D	7.	J
3.	H	8.	C
4.	I	9.	F
5.	B	10.	A

Learning Outcomes

1. Cyanosis is bluish discoloration of the skin and mucous membranes.
2. The dermis regulates body temperature by dilating and constricting capillaries, and it transmits messages via nerve endings to the CNS.
3. Three types of glands in the skin are sebaceous (oil), eccrine sweat glands, and apocrine sweat glands.
4. A vesicle is an elevated, fluid-filled, round- or oval-shaped, palpable mass with thin, translucent walls and circumscribed borders. Vesicles are smaller than 0.5 cm.
5. Keloids occur from a scar related to surgery or ear piercing. It is an elevated, irregular, darkened area of excess scar tissue caused by excessive collagen formation during healing. There is a higher incidence of keloids in people of African descent.
6. Clubbing is an angle of the nail base that is greater than 180 degrees.
7. A biopsy is done when a sample of a nodule or skin is needed to rule out malignancy. It can be done with a syringe to pull out fluid, or with a special biopsy instrument.

8. A culture and sensitivity (C&S) is done when fluid obtained from a pustule or abscess is thought to have a bacterial or viral infection.

9. Suspected allergens are applied to normal skin under patches. Reactions range from weak with redness or itching, to strong with pain and blisters.

10. Alopecia is hair loss.

Apply What You Learned

1. A wheal would be present and must be a certain size in order to characterize it as positive. A wheal is an elevated, often reddish area with an irregular border caused by diffuse fluid in tissues rather than free fluid in a cavity, as in vesicles. Size will vary.

Multiple Choice

1.	C	6.	C	11.	A
2.	D	7.	A	12.	A
3.	A	8.	D	13.	C
4.	B	9.	D	14.	B
5.	C	10.	B	15.	C

Chapter 45 Caring for Clients With Skin Disorders

Matching

1.	F	6.	H
2.	J	7.	I
3.	D	8.	A
4.	G	9.	E
5.	B	10.	C

Learning Outcomes

1. Psoriasis is a chronic, noninfectious skin disorder. It is characterized by raised, reddened, round circumscribed plaques of varied size, covered by silvery-white scales.

2. Contact dermatitis is caused by a hypersensitivity response or a chemical irritation. Major sources include: perfumes, dyes, plants, metals, and chemicals.

3. Cellulitis is a localized infection of the dermis and subcutaneous tissue. It can occur following a wound or skin ulcer.

4. Folliculitis begins at the skin surface and extends down into the hair follicle. It is most often caused by *Staphylococcus aureus*. The bacteria release enzymes and chemical agents that cause an inflammation.

5. Basal cell carcinoma is a slow-growing cancer that usually appears on sun-exposed areas of the body, such as the head and neck. These carcinomas can recur in the same location after treatment. They have a shiny, pearly white, or pink appearance in nodular carcinoma. The superficial carcinomas are a flat papule that is often red.

6. Steps to prevent sking cancer include the following: minimize exposure to the sun between the hours of 10 a.m. and 4 p.m. when the ultraviolet rays are the strongest; wear a wide-brimmed hat, sunglasses, and a long woven shirt; use sunscreen and remember to reapply; and avoid tanning booths.

7. Pressure ulcers are ischemic lesions of the skin and underlying tissue caused by external pressure that impairs the flow of blood and lymph. The ischemia causes tissue necrosis and eventual ulceration.

8. Pressure ulcer stages are as follows: Stage I is nonblanchable erythema of intact skin. Stage II is partial-thickness loss. Stage III is full-thickness loss involving damage of subcutaneous tissue. Stage IV is full-thickness skin loss with extensive destruction and tissue necrosis with possible sinus tracts.

9. Melanoma is a skin cancer that causes 4% of all skin cancer cases. The incidence is highest in Caucasians, people who had severe, blistering sunburns during childhood, and in people who live in sunny climates, burn easily, and visit tanning booths. They also may arise from lesions that are already present or from skin that is normally covered with clothing. Melanomas start off flat, but with progression into the lymph, they become raised.

10. Nevi are moles and the precursor for the development of melanoma.

Apply What You Learned

1. To self-screen for sking cancer, the client follows the ABCD rule: A is for asymmetry of the mole; B is for border irregularity; C is for color variation; D is for diameter greater than 5mm.

2. This client presented with basal cell carcinoma.

3. The client should wear sunscreen even in the tanning booth. She should try to avoid the sun between 10 a.m. and 4 p.m. as well as avoid the tanning beds. The client should wear wide-brimmed hats and sunglasses. She should also protect exposed arms and legs with woven clothing.

Multiple Choice

1.	A	6.	D	11.	B
2.	B	7.	A	12.	A
3.	C	8.	C	13.	C
4.	C	9.	B	14.	A
5.	C	10.	C	15.	C

Chapter 46 Caring for Clients With Burns

Matching

1.	F	6.	H
2.	D	7.	J
3.	G	8.	B
4.	I	9.	C
5.	A	10.	E

Learning Outcomes

1. Burns are an injury in which a transfer of energy from a heat source to the human body results in tissue loss, damage, or irreversible destruction.
2. The "rule of nines" is a rapid method of estimating the extent of burns. It is used during prehospital and emergency care phases.
3. Curling's ulcer is an acute ulceration of the stomach or duodenum that may form following a burn injury.
4. Debridement is the process of removing dead tissue from the wound.
5. Initial assessments regarding burns include: time of injury, cause, first-aid treatment, past medical history, age, medications, and body weight.
6. Nursing diagnoses related to the burn client include: Deficient Fluid Volume, Risk for Infection, Impaired Physical Mobility, Acute Pain, and Powerlessness.
7. A contracture is a permanent shortening of connective tissue.
8. Silver nitrate is a bacteriostatic agent that inhibits many different gram-positive and gram-negative organisms. It is used as a 0.5% solution in distilled water to prevent burn wound infections.
9. Urinalysis, CBC, serum electrolytes, total protein and albumin, ABGs, pulse oximetry, CXR, and ECGs are tests done to monitor and assess burns.
10. A full-thickness burn is a third degree burn that involves all layers of skin.

Apply What You Learned

1. 4 ½% of his body is burned. Remember that the rule of nines is just an estimate.
2. Silvadene would be used on this client to prevent burn wound infections. This client may also see a plastic surgeon throughout the healing process to identify if corrective surgery is needed.

Multiple Choice

1. C	6. B	11. D
2. D	7. A	12. A
3. C	8. A	13. B
4. C	9. C	14. D
5. A	10. A	15. C

Chapter 47 Mental Health and Assessment

Matching

1. D	6. G
2. F	7. I
3. A	8. B
4. C	9. J
5. H	10. E

Learning Outcomes

1. Aspects of a mentally healthy person are: an accurate assessment of reality, healthy self-concept, ability to relate to others, sense of meaning in life, creativity/productivity, control over one's behavior, and an adaptability to change and conflict.
2. Insight is self-understanding.
3. Neurotransmitters include acetylcholine, dopamine, norepinephrine, serotonin, and GABA.
4. A synapse is the space between the axon and its target cell's dendrite.
5. Stigma is the negative attitude that marks people who have certain conditions as less valuable.
6. Psychologic functions include: thinking, feeling, behavior, responses to situations, relationships, and community support.
7. Four aspects of self-concept are body image, role performance, identity, and self-esteem.
8. The five most common mental illnesses are: major depressive disorder, ETOH abuse, schizophrenia, self-inflicted injuries, and bipolar disorder.
9. Mental illnesses are diagnosed according to the diagnostic criteria published in the *Diagnostic and Statistical Manual of Mental Disorders*.
10. Concrete thinking is literal and without creativity.

Apply What You Learned

1. Elements of a complete mental status assessment are: appearance, orientation to surroundings, mood and affect, speech, thoughts, hallucinations, behavior, memory, and judgment.
2. "What happened that caused you to come to the hospital?" It is straightforward and nonjudgmental.

Multiple Choice

1.	B	6.	D	11.	A
2.	B	7.	C	12.	C
3.	C	8.	B	13.	D
4.	A	9.	A	14.	A
5.	D	10.	C	15.	B

Chapter 48 Caring for Clients With Cognitive Disorders

Matching

1.	J	6.	H
2.	B	7.	D
3.	I	8.	G
4.	A	9.	E
5.	C	10.	F

Learning Outcomes

1. Normal memory lapses may include forgetting where you left your keys or wallet, searching to find a word that is on the tip of your tongue, and losing track of what you planned to say.
2. Delirium may manifest either with motor agitation or motor retardation, sudden onset of severe agitation and hallucinations, or declining level of consciousness progressing to coma.
3. The MMSE consists of questions related to orientation, registration, attention and calculation, recall, and language, for a total score of thirty points.
4. Agnosia is the loss of comprehension of visual, auditory, or other sensations, although the sensory structures are intact.
5. Common causes of dementia include: neurodegenerative disorders, vascular-based disorders, metabolic diseases, immunologic diseases, infections, tumors, and seizures.
6. Alzheimer's disease is a neurologic disorder in which neurofibrillary tangles and beta-amyloid plaques cause deterioration of brain function, characterized by a progressive loss of memory.
7. Risk factors for vascular dementia include advanced age, hypertension, hyperlipidemia, atrial fibrillation, coronary artery disease, and diabetes.
8. Delirium has a quick onset, is worse at night, includes sleep disturbances, and is temporary. Dementia has a gradual onset and symptoms progress slowly. The client frequently awakens in the night. It is chronic with a life expectancy after diagnosis of eight years.
9. Hyperorality is a condition in which clients will put anything within reach into their mouths.
10. Medications used to treat dementia are: Aricept, Exelon, Razadyne, Namenda, and Cognex.

Apply What You Learned

1. The above characteristics indicates onset of Alzheimer's disease.
2. After a definite diagnosis, the client should be started on medication to slow the progression of dementia. Senior centers, home nurses, and perhaps a meals-on-wheels program would be beneficial for this client. A senior center might ensure the client is socially active and not becoming withdrawn. Home care nurses can make certain the client is taking medication and is safe at home, and Meals-on-Wheels can ensure the client has an appropriate diet.
3. Nursing diagnoses for this client would include: Risk for Injury related to impaired judgment and disorientation, Disturbed Thought Processes, Language Deficit, and Deficient Knowledge.

Multiple Choice

1. B	6. D	11. C
2. D	7. A	12. B
3. A	8. B	13. B
4. C	9. D	14. A
5. C	10. D	15. D

Matching

1.	C	6.	F
2.	B	7.	I
3.	J	8.	D
4.	A	9.	H
5.	E	10.	G

Learning Outcomes

1. Psychosis refers to a thought disorder that causes the following symptoms: delusions, hallucinations, disorganized speech, and disorganized behavior.
2. A hallucination is a sensory experience that seems real to the client but is not related to external stimuli. The most common hallucinations are auditory; the second most common are visual. Hallucinations can involve any of the senses.
3. The four types of cognitive impairments are: attention, executive function, awareness of the illness, and short-term memory.
4. Affect is the nonverbal expression of emotion.
5. Milieu therapy is an environment in which therapy is provided for clients with psychoses.
6. Nursing diagnoses for clients with psychotic disorders include: Risk for Violence, Disturbed Thought Processes, Ineffective Coping, and Impaired Social Interaction.
7. Outcomes for a client with schizophrenia include: cause no harm to self or others, have reality-based thinking, use healthy coping skills, take medications regularly, and keep in touch with family and friends.
8. Tardive dyskinesia is the late onset of abnormal movement. It is an extrapyramidal effect that develops after extended antipsychotic drug therapy.
9. During the prodromal phase, the client has early symptoms before a full psychotic episode.
10. A client with bizarre delusions believes clearly improbable ideas that are not derived from real-life experiences.

Apply What You Learned

1. This client might receive a diagnosis of schizophrenia.
2. Only one person should interact with the client at a time to prevent overstimulation. Keep environmental noise to a minimum and do not speak loudly. This will enable the client to concentrate on your voice and differentiate real stimuli from the non-real stimuli. Initially ask about the hallucination so that a determination can be made if there is an intent to commit harm. Focus on reality. Do not ask the client to continually describe the hallucination. Bring the client back to reality as often as necessary without getting the client agitated. Do not argue with the client's experience. Reassure the client that he or she is safe. Share your own perceptions

by letting the client know that you do not hear any voices. Avoid touching the client if the client is actively hallucinating. The client may see this as a threat, and the goal is safety for the client and staff.

Multiple Choice

1.	C	6.	D	11.	A
2.	A	7.	C	12.	B
3.	B	8.	B	13.	D
4.	B	9.	A	14.	A
5.	D	10.	A	15.	A

Chapter 50 Caring for Clients With Mood Disorders

Matching

1.	D	6.	B
2.	C	7.	E
3.	A	8.	F
4.	G	9.	J
5.	H	10.	I

Learning Outcomes

1. Mood is a pervasive and sustained emotion that influences how a person perceives the world.
2. Risk factors for depression include: family history, female gender, stressful life events, substance abuse, postpartum period, chronic medical condition, and history of a suicide attempt.
3. Psychomotor agitation is an increase in activity.
4. Protective factors for suicide are: effective and appropriate clinical care, easy access to support, family support, and learned skills in problem solving and conflict resolution.
5. Suicide is the taking of one's own life.
6. Anticholinergic side effects include: dry mouth, increased heart rate, constipation, pupil dilation, blurred near vision, dry eyes, and photophobia.
7. Foods to avoid when taking MAOIs include: aged cheese, preserved meats, liver, draft beer, soy sauce, yeast, and caffeine.
8. ECT is the application of electrical current to the brain, which induces a generalized seizure.
9. While manic, the client feels elated, euphoric, high, or unusually good. People in a manic episode frequently lack insight about their illness and its effects on themselves and others. They often resist treatment and sometimes require involuntary hospitalization. Periods of mania alternate with periods of depression.
10. Side effects of lithium include fine hand tremors, weight gain, nausea, slurred speech, mental confusion, decreased urine output, and sometimes coma or death.

Apply What You Learned

1. Use open-ended questions when asking the client to express feelings. Clarify the client's statements. Gather data for assessment and validate the client's feelings. Obtain a "no self-harm" contract and assess the client's current safety.
2. "Are you thinking about hurting yourself?"

Multiple Choice

1.	B	6.	A	11.	A
2.	A	7.	C	12.	B
3.	C	8.	B	13.	C
4.	D	9.	D	14.	A
5.	D	10.	C	15.	D

Chapter 51 Caring for Clients With Anxiety Disorders

Matching

1.	C	6.	A
2.	I	7.	H
3.	B	8.	F
4.	J	9.	G
5.	E	10.	D

Learning Outcomes

1. Anxiety is a feeling of uneasiness and activation of the ANS in response to a vague, nonspecific threat.
2. Manifestations of anxiety attacks include: palpitations, sweating, trembling, feeling of choking, chest pain, nausea, feeling dizzy, and fear of losing control.
3. PTSD is a debilitating condition that follows an extreme traumatic stressor such as a violent personal attack or war.
4. Medical conditions associated with anxiety are: hypoglycemia, asthma, COPD, B12 deficiency, hyperthyroidism, and neoplasms.
5. Paradoxical responses are contradictory or opposite, so the client's response is the opposite of what is expected from a medication.
6. Resilience is the quality of being hardy or "stress resistant." Resilient people are perceived as able to cope and flourish despite stress.
7. Anti-anxiety agents include: Xanax, Librium, Klonopin, Valium, Ativan, Serax, and Tranxene.
8. A phobia is a persistent and irrational fear.
9. OCD is characterized by compulsions or obsessions, which the affected person recognizes are excessive or unreasonable. The obsessions or compulsions cause marked distress and take more than one hour each day, or significantly interfere with the person's life.
10. Coping behaviors are ways to adapt to or manage stress or change.

Apply What You Learned

1. The nurse would expect a diagnosis of posttraumatic stress disorder.
2. This client would benefit from learning coping techniques, cognitive-behavioral therapy, promoting resilience, and the use of medication and regular therapy sessions with a licensed professional.

Multiple Choice

1.	A	6.	B	11.	A
2.	C	7.	C	12.	D
3.	C	8.	C	13.	A
4.	D	9.	D	14.	B
5.	B	10.	D	15.	C

Chapter 52 Caring for Clients With Personality Disorders

Matching

1.	C	6.	E
2.	D	7.	I
3.	G	8.	J
4.	H	9.	F
5.	B	10.	A

Learning Outcomes

1. Personality is the relatively stable way in which a person thinks, feels, and behaves.
2. Cluster A is odd and eccentric. Cluster B is dramatic and emotional, and Cluster C is anxiety- and fear-based.
3. Inappropriate affect occurs when the client has an emotional response that is not culturally appropriate for the situation, such as laughing when someone's pet dies.
4. APD is a pervasive pattern of disregarding and violating the rights of others.
5. A narcissistic person has a need for admiration, patterns of grandiosity, and lack of empathy for others. They have an inflated sense of self and feel entitled.
6. Clients with dependent personality disorder have a need to be taken care of. They have submissive and clinging behavior. They have difficulty making everyday decisions without help and advice from others.
7. Coping mechanisms for a client who suffers from self-harm are: talk to someone, delay your decision for five minutes, call a crisis line, yell, scream, cry, sing loudly, or pound on your bed until you are exhausted.
8. Borderline personality disorder describes clients who are on the border between anxiety and psychosis.
9. Parasuicidal behavior is behavior aimed at harming but not killing oneself.
10. Ideas of reference are the misinterpretation of everyday events, believing that these events have personal meaning for them.

Apply What You Learned

1. Make the unit rules clear. Policies must be maintained. Stick to the rules consistently. Include the client in problem solving and have a conference with him or her. Remember who is the client and who is the professional.

Multiple Choice

1. C	6. D	11. A
2. B	7. C	12. B
3. A	8. B	13. A
4. A	9. C	14. A
5. A	10. C	15. C

Chapter 53 Caring for Clients With Substance Abuse or Dependency

Matching

1. G	6. A
2. H	7. C
3. F	8. E
4. I	9. D
5. J	10. B

Learning Outcomes

1. Denial is the refusal to acknowledge the existence of a real situation or feelings.
2. Commonly abused substances include: alcohol, opioids, sedatives, cocaine, hallucinogens, inhalants, caffeine, and nicotine.
3. Someone withdrawing from alcohol may have elevated vital signs, anxiety, tremors, diaphoresis, slurred speech, GI disturbances, and disorientation.
4. Korsakoff's syndrome is a group of symptoms caused by a deficiency in the B vitamins, including thiamine, riboflavin, and folic acid.
5. Wernicke's syndrome is characterized by ataxia, paralysis of the eye muscles, and mental confusion. It is the result of severe vitamin B1 deficiency from lack of adequate nutritional intake.
6. Fetal alcohol syndrome presents with low birth weight, small head circumference, facial anomalies, and neurodevelopmental disorders.
7. Detoxification is the removal of a substance from the body.
8. Rehabilitation is a continuous phase related to substance abuse. Medications and therapies, as well as support groups, are utilized to prevent relapses for the rest of the client's life. The goals of rehab are to maintain sobriety, develop new coping skills, make a plan for relapse prevention and living life with all responsibilities, and be able to cope effectively.
9. Dual diagnosis refers to someone who is diagnosed with a substance use disorder and a serious mental illness.

10. An impaired nurse is someone who is working under the influence of substances. They may exhibit mood changes, irritability, forgetfulness, isolation from co-workers, and work performance may suffer.

Apply What You Learned

1. Stereotypes related to alcoholics include: lack of education, low socioeconomic background, non-Caucasian ethnicity, and unemployed. Everyone, regardless of status and position in life, is susceptible to alcoholism.
2. The student nurse would begin by asking clients how much and how often they drink. They will also ask if clients use any nonprescribed drugs and for what purpose. The student nurse also needs to ask what these substances do for them. Does the client get high or relaxed? Also, try to identify any problems the client has been having since using any substance. Find out the last time they used, and what was the substance of choice.

Multiple Choice

1.	C	6.	C	11.	D
2.	B	7.	C	12.	A
3.	D	8.	B	13.	C
4.	A	9.	C	14.	C
5.	A	10.	D	15.	D